Methods for Analysing and Reporting EQ-5D Data

Nancy Devlin · David Parkin · Bas Janssen

Methods for Analysing and Reporting EQ-5D Data

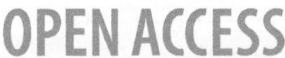

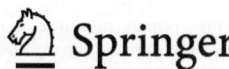

Nancy Devlin
Centre for Health Policy
University of Melbourne
Melbourne, Australia

David Parkin
Office of Health Economics
London, UK

Bas Janssen
EuroQol Research Foundation
Rotterdam, The Netherlands

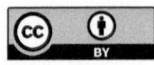

ISBN 978-3-030-47624-3   ISBN 978-3-030-47622-9   (eBook)
https://doi.org/10.1007/978-3-030-47622-9

This Springer imprint is published by the registered company Springer Nature Switzerland AG
The registered company address is: Gewerbestrasse 11, 6330 Cham, Switzerland

Foreword By Niek Klazinga

Efforts to capture health and healthcare outcomes through measurement—at personal, group and population level—have been around for many years. In the broad field of today's patient reported measurement instruments, the generic EQ-5D instruments to capture health status stand out for their use over three decades and have been implemented and used for a variety of purposes. These include the systematic assessment of health of populations, both cross-sectionally and over time, (economic) evaluation of health interventions and, more recently, as a supportive tool in the strive towards value-based health care. This means that users may vary from patient and clinicians towards all stakeholders in the healthcare system that seek to underpin their decisions with aggregated patient reported information, such as healthcare managers, financiers and policymakers.

Although a lot of literature has become available over the years on the validity and reliability of the various EQ-5D instruments, general information about how to analyse the data once collected, is scarce and scattered. This book seeks to fill this void and will prove to be a welcome support for all parties who want to analyse the collected data. After a concise explanation of the existing instruments, the reader will find detailed information on data analyses related to topics like the EQ VAS, the calculation and use of EQ-5D values and analyses of EQ-5D data for specific purposes.

With the broadening of the use of generic PROMs to include day to day management of health care and creating more value in the healthcare system, a new audience will start exploring its use. For all users this book will provide support in determining whether for them the EQ-5D instruments are 'fit for use' and how collected data can best be analysed.

Since 2017 the Organization for Economic Cooperation and Development (OECD) has started the Patient Reported Indicator Survey program (PaRIS) to support member states in strengthening a data-driven shift towards value-based healthcare systems. The EQ-5D instruments and the related expertise that has been gained over the years play an important role in this endeavour.

This book can help to turn enthusiasm of collecting data on PROMs into an evidence based and well-informed analysis of the aggregated findings for local, national as well as international comparative use.

Niek Klazinga, M.D. Ph.D.
Strategic Lead Healthcare Quality
and Outcomes Program OECD
Paris, France

Professor of Social Medicine
Amsterdam University Medical Centre, AMC
Amsterdam, Netherlands

Foreword By Elly Stolk and Gouke Bonsel

When the authors informed us of the plans for this book about EQ-5D, we were immediately excited by its potential to support users in their analysis and reporting of EQ-5D data.

The EQ-5D is a very widely used measure of self-reported health globally. It is a concise, generic questionnaire which is accompanied by value sets, and this has made it particularly widely used in economic evaluation. EQ-5D use is supported by the availability of a wide range of language versions. The EQ-5D 'family' of instruments has expanded to include both three- and five-level versions and a version suitable for use in children, with further instruments planned or in development. User guides are available to support and guide data collection.

However, to date, there has been no comprehensive source of advice to users on the methods that can be applied to analyse EQ-5D data. This book addresses that gap, providing users for the first time with detailed explanation of methods for analysing and reporting EQ-5D data.

One of the main messages in this book is the rich and detailed insights that can be obtained by analysing all aspects of the EQ-5D data provided by respondents. The EQ-5D is unique, as a generic patient reported outcomes questionnaire, in yielding respondents' self-reported descriptions of their own health; value sets which can be used to summarise those descriptions; and a self-assessed measure of overall health, the visual analogue scale (EQ VAS). Each of these elements provides important data, with different properties, that require different methods of analysis and provide different insights.

Economic evaluation of healthcare interventions was the primary field of application for which the EQ-5D developers envisaged the instrument to be useful, and its uptake in this field has made EQ-5D mainstream since its inception. For two decades now, market decisions on pharmaceuticals have relied heavily on the seemingly simple numbers of EQ-5D values. However, even in this context, where the focus is on the use of value sets to estimate QALYs, the full analysis of patients' profile and EQ VAS data can enrich an understanding of patients' health problems and improvements in health from treatment.

Beyond economic evaluation, there are expanding uses of EQ-5D. It has long been used in population health surveys, for example. More recently, the collection of Patient Reported Outcomes Measures (PROMs) has emerged as a major field of application of EQ-5D. The 'PROMification' of healthcare systems reflects a deeply felt need for accountability and quality improvement. In this context, the collection of PROMs such as EQ-5D is at the core of a movement aiming at quality improvement. While not developed for this use, EQ-5D earned a position as primary candidate for PROMs in this setting, due to its brevity and the ample evidence available about its validity as a generic measure of health. Notably, while EQ-5D PROMs data can be analysed by applying value sets, the rationale for doing so is not clear. This broader application of EQ-5D implies a broader and appropriate set of metrics. Increased use of EQ-5D as a PROM has stressed the need for considering what we can learn from the data captured in the EQ-5D descriptive system, but guidance on how to analyse this data has been lacking. It is therefore particularly timely that authors Nancy Devlin, David Parkin and Bas Janssen provide a comprehensive set of methods that can be applied to analyse and report patients' EQ-5D responses in this context.

This book marks the start of a new phase in EQ-5D applications and analysis. We hope the reader feels as inspired as we did when reading the book.

Elly Stolk, Ph.D.
Scientific Team Leader

Founding EuroQol Member
EuroQol Research Foundation
Rotterdam, The Netherlands

Gouke Bonsel, M.D. Ph.D.
Founding EuroQol Member
EuroQol Research Foundation
Rotterdam, The Netherlands

Preface

The EQ-5D is a short questionnaire designed to measure patient reported health in a broad, 'generic' manner. Its strength lies both in its brevity; and the ability to measure patient health in a manner that can be compared across patients, diseases and treatments. Since its development nearly three decades ago, it has become the most widely used Patient Reported Outcomes questionnaire internationally, used in population health surveys, clinical studies and in routine outcomes measurement in healthcare systems (Devlin and Brooks 2017).

Yet, despite nearly 30 years of its use, there is no comprehensive guide to users on how to analyse EQ-5D data. The EuroQol group, which developed the EQ-5D, provides users guides, but these have as their emphasis an explanation of the questionnaire and how to collect the data, rather than how to analyse it. We frequently receive requests for advice on how to analyse EQ-5D data, once collected.

Our aim in writing this book is to fill this need by providing clear and comprehensive guidance on the methods which can be used to analyse EQ-5D data. In doing so, we set out to encourage users to make full use of the data collected from patients, in order to maximise the insights that can be obtained. Our intended audience is both new users of the EQ-5D, who may not be familiar with how to analyse the data, and experienced analysts, as a reminder that simple descriptive analysis can yield powerful insights that should precede and inform more sophisticated modelling.

In each chapter, we explain the methods in a straightforward way, with a focus on the underlying measurement properties of the EQ-5D instruments and how that affects the way to approach data analysis. Understanding the nature of the various distinctive elements of data generated by the EQ-5D (the profile, the EQ VAS and the EQ-5D values) is critical, and our focus is on the intuition underlying each approach. We have not set out to write a statistics textbook, so where appropriate we refer readers to appropriate sources for further information.

In order to encourage users to use the methods we describe here, this book will be accompanied by code in the most widely used statistical software: STATA, R, SAS, SPSS and where possible, excel. That code will be free to download and will be available from the EuroQol Group website: www.euroqol.org.

We hope you find this book useful!

Nancy Devlin
Professor of Heath Economics
University of Melbourne
Melbourne, Australia

Senior Visiting Fellow
Office of Health Economics
London, UK

David Parkin
Senior Visiting Fellow
Office of Health Economics
London, UK

Honorary Visiting Professor, City
University of London
London, UK

Bas Janssen
Senior Scientist, EuroQol Research Foundation
Rotterdam, The Netherlands

Acknowledgements

The authors are grateful to Yan Feng, Bernarda Zamora, Mark Oppe, Sarah Dewilde, Eleanor Pullenayegum, Ning Yan Gu and Allan Wailoo for their contribution of examples for this book, and to Amy Livingstone for her assistance with seeking copyright permissions. Mike Herdman and Bram Roudijk provided helpful comments on earlier drafts. Funding to write this book was received from the EuroQol Research Foundation. Views expressed in the book are those of the authors and are not necessarily those of the EuroQol Research Foundation.

Contents

About the Authors

Prof. Nancy Devlin is Professor of Health Economics and Director of the Centre for Health Policy at the University of Melbourne, Australia, and Senior Visiting Fellow at the Office of Health Economics, London. She is President of ISPOR (2019–2020) and past president of the EuroQol Group. Her principal areas of research are the measurement and valuation of Patient Reported Outcomes; and the cost effectiveness thresholds used in making judgments about value for money in health care. Previous books include 'Economic Analysis in Health Care', 'Using Patient Reported Outcomes to Improve Health Care', and 'EQ-5D Valuation Sets: An Inventory, Comparative Review and User Guide'.

Prof. David Parkin is Visiting Professor of Health Economics at City, University of London, and Senior Visiting Fellow at the Office of Health Economics, London. He has been a member of the EuroQol group for over 20 years and was one of the developers of the EQ-5D-5L. He has published extensively on the EQ-5D as well as other topics in health economics and health status measurement. This includes a popular textbook on health economics, 'Economic Analysis in Health Care' with Stephen Morris, Nancy Devlin and Ann Spencer, and the handbook 'Using Patient Reported Outcomes To Improve Health Care', with John Appleby and Nancy Devlin.

Dr. Bas Janssen is an independent researcher and consultant in health economics and outcomes research. He is a senior scientist at the business office of the EuroQol Research Foundation and affiliated to the Erasmus University Medical Center in Rotterdam. He specialises in the measurement and valuation of Patient Reported Outcomes, psychometrics and biostatistics. He has published extensively on EQ-5D, including the handbook 'Self-Reported Population Health: An International Perspective based on EQ-5D' with Agota Szende and Juan Cabasés.

Chapter 1
An Introduction to EQ-5D Instruments and Their Applications

The aims of this chapter are

- to introduce the EQ-5D 'family' of questionnaires: what they are for, how they are used and what they measure;
- to explain the nature of the data that the EQ-5D questionnaires generate and how that affects the way that EQ-5D data should be analysed;
- to examine how the purposes for which EQ-5D data are collected affect the ways that they should be analysed and reported; and
- to describe good practice in data handling and preparing for statistical analysis of EQ-5D data.

Our focus, throughout this book, is on the analysis of EQ-5D data. The book is designed to meet the needs of those who have, or are planning to collect, EQ-5D data. Our hope is that this book will encourage all analysts, both those new to the EQ-5D and those experienced in using EQ-5D questionnaires, to make full use of the data provided by respondents, and to maximise the insights possible from those data.

It is also important to say what this book does not address. We do not provide guidance on methods of Patient Reported Outcome (PRO) data collection or PRO study design. For such guidance, you may wish to consult resources such as the SPIRIT-PRO[1] guidelines on inclusion of PROs in clinical trials (Calvert et al. 2018), the United States Food and Drug Administration (FDA) guidance to industry on the use of PRO measures in evidence to support labelling claims (FDA 2009); the European Medicines Agency (EMA) guidance regarding use of health-related quality of life (HRQoL) in labelling studies (EMA 2006); and the various good practice guidelines published by the International Society for Pharmacoeconomics & Outcomes Research (ISPOR), for example on electronic PROs (Zbrozek et al. 2013), and on collection of PROs in paediatric studies (Matza et al. 2013). Also, we do not offer

---

[1]SPIRIT: Standard Protocol Items: Recommendations for Interventional Trials.

guidance on which EQ-5D questionnaire to use in what circumstances—for example, in what populations to use the youth version of the EQ-5D (the EQ-5D-Y); whether to use the three- or five-level version; and how and when to use the paper, telephone, proxy or digital versions. Information on these Issues is provided in the User Guides available online at: www.euroqol.org.

A glossary of the EQ-5D terms used in this and subsequent chapters is in an appendix.

1.1 Measuring Health Using the EQ-5D

The EQ-5D is a concise, generic measure of self-reported health which is accompanied by weights reflecting the relative importance to people of different types of health problems. The concept of health being measured by EQ-5D is variously described as health status or HRQoL,[2] the latter of which might be defined as:

> The value assigned to duration of life as modified by the impairments, functional status, perceptions and social opportunities that are influenced by disease, injury, treatment or policy. (Patrick and Erickson 1993)

The EQ-5D is 'generic' because it measures health in a way that can be compared across different sorts of patients, disease areas, and treatments. The researchers who developed it—the EuroQol Group—aimed to develop a questionnaire which was brief, minimised the burden of data collection, and could be used in a wide variety of health care sector applications (Devlin and Brooks 2017). The '5D' in its name refers to its use of 5 dimensions for describing health states: Mobility, Usual Activities, Self-care, Pain & Discomfort and Anxiety & Depression. In the original EQ-5D questionnaire (Fig. 1.1), now known as the EQ-5D-3L, three levels of problems are described in each dimension, representing no, moderate, or extreme problems in the Pain & Discomfort and Anxiety & Depression dimensions and no, some, and inability to in the Mobility, Usual Activities and Self-care dimensions.[3] In the more recent EQ-5D-5L (Fig. 1.2), the number of levels has been expanded from three to five and these are explicitly expressed as no, mild, moderate, severe and extreme or unable to (Herdman et al. 2011). A version of the instrument, the EQ-5D-Y (Fig. 1.3), has been developed for young people and children, retaining the same five dimensions (Wille et al. 2010).

In each case, the questionnaires are designed mainly for self-completion, either by people who are receiving treatment (for example patients in a clinical trial) or people in other settings (for example a sample of the general public in a population health survey). (As well as the self-report questionnaire, there are also 'interview'

---

[2]For a discussion of definitional and conceptual issues relating to HRQOL, see Morris et al. (2012), Sect. 11.3.

[3]For the Mobility dimension the worst level is 'confined to bed'.

MOBILITY

I have no problems in walking about   ❑

I have some problems in walking about   ❑

I am confined to bed   ❑

SELF-CARE

I have no problems with self-care   ❑

I have some problems washing or dressing myself   ❑

I am unable to wash or dress myself   ❑

USUAL ACTIVITIES (*e.g. work, study, housework, family or leisure activities*)

I have no problems with performing my usual activities   ❑

I have some problems with performing my usual activities   ❑

I am unable to perform my usual activities   ❑

PAIN / DISCOMFORT

I have no pain or discomfort   ❑

I have moderate pain or discomfort   ❑

I have extreme pain or discomfort   ❑

ANXIETY / DEPRESSION

I am not anxious or depressed   ❑

I am moderately anxious or depressed   ❑

I am extremely anxious or depressed   ❑

Fig. 1.1 EQ-5D-3L descriptive system. *Source* EuroQol Research Foundation. *EQ-5D-3L User Guide, 2018.* Latest version available from: https://euroqol.org/publications/user-guides

and 'proxy' versions, designed for special cases where people whose EQ-5D data are being collected cannot complete a self-report questionnaire themselves.) For this reason, the EQ-5D belongs to a category of questionnaires often referred to as PROs and sometimes as Patient Reported Outcome Measures (PROMs). PROs aim to measure people's subjective assessment of their own health in a manner that is systematic, valid and reliable. There is growing recognition that such data from

Under each heading, please tick the ONE box that best describes your health TODAY.

MOBILITY

I have no problems in walking about ☐
I have slight problems in walking about ☐
I have moderate problems in walking about ☐
I have severe problems in walking about ☐
I am unable to walk about ☐

SELF-CARE

I have no problems washing or dressing myself ☐
I have slight problems washing or dressing myself ☐
I have moderate problems washing or dressing myself ☐
I have severe problems washing or dressing myself ☐
I am unable to wash or dress myself ☐

USUAL ACTIVITIES (*e.g. work, study, housework, family or leisure activities*)

I have no problems doing my usual activities ☐
I have slight problems doing my usual activities ☐
I have moderate problems doing my usual activities ☐
I have severe problems doing my usual activities ☐
I am unable to do my usual activities ☐

PAIN / DISCOMFORT

I have no pain or discomfort ☐
I have slight pain or discomfort ☐
I have moderate pain or discomfort ☐
I have severe pain or discomfort ☐
I have extreme pain or discomfort ☐

ANXIETY / DEPRESSION

I am not anxious or depressed ☐
I am slightly anxious or depressed ☐
I am moderately anxious or depressed ☐
I am severely anxious or depressed ☐
I am extremely anxious or depressed ☐

Fig. 1.2 EQ-5D-5L descriptive system. *Source* EuroQol Research Foundation. *EQ-5D-5L User Guide, 2019*. Latest version available from: https://euroqol.org/publications/user-guides

Under each heading, please tick the ONE box that best describes your health TODAY

Mobility *(walking about)*

I have <u>no</u> problems walking about ❑

I have <u>some</u> problems walking about ❑

I have <u>a lot</u> of problems walking about ❑

Looking after myself

I have <u>no</u> problems washing or dressing myself ❑

I have <u>some</u> problems washing or dressing myself ❑

I have <u>a lot</u> of problems washing or dressing myself ❑

Doing usual activities *(for example, going to school, hobbies, sports, playing, doing things with family or friends)*

I have <u>no</u> problems doing my usual activities ❑

I have <u>some</u> problems doing my usual activities ❑

I have <u>a lot</u> of problems doing my usual activities ❑

Having pain or discomfort

I have <u>no</u> pain or discomfort ❑

I have <u>some</u> pain or discomfort ❑

I have <u>a lot</u> of pain or discomfort ❑

Feeling worried, sad or unhappy

I am <u>not</u> worried, sad or unhappy ❑

I am <u>a bit</u> worried, sad or unhappy ❑

I am <u>very</u> worried, sad or unhappy ❑

Fig. 1.3 EQ-5D-Y. *Source* EuroQol Research Foundation. *EQ-5D-Y User Guide, 2014.* Latest version available from: https://euroqol.org/publications/user-guides

patients provides important information that complements the clinical endpoints traditionally used in medical care, and can pick up problems and issues missed by them (Appleby et al. 2015). For example, Robert Temple from the FDA stated that "The use of Patient Reported Outcome instruments is part of a general movement toward the idea that the patient, properly queried, is the best source of information about how he or she feels" (Bren 2006). The EQ-5D is one of the most widely used PRO measures internationally, and by 2016 the EQ-5D-3L was available in 176 language versions the EQ-5D-5L 123 and the EQ-5D-Y 40 (Devlin and Brooks 2017).

The EQ-5D questionnaire comprises two parts. The first is the EQ-5D descriptive system, as shown in Figs. 1.1, 1.2, and 1.3. Respondents are asked to tick boxes to indicate the level of problem they experience on each of the five dimensions. The combination of these ticks under each dimension describes that person's EQ-5D self-reported health state, often called an 'EQ-5D profile', which is described in more detail below.

The second part of the questionnaire is the EQ VAS, so called because it incorporates a Visual Analogue Scale. This captures the respondent's overall assessment of their health on a scale from 0 (worst health imaginable) to 100 (best health imaginable). The current versions of the EQ-5D-3L and 5L use the same EQ VAS, shown in Fig. 1.4, but the original version of the 3L had a slightly different format, as does the EQ-5D-Y.

The EQ-5D profile data can also be supplemented by using a 'scoring' or 'weighting' system to convert profile data to a single number—EQ-5D values. These scoring systems are usually based on preferences—that is, the problems on each dimension are weighted to reflect how good or bad people think they are. So, for example, many studies have shown that problems with pain and discomfort often carry more weight than problems with self-care as reported by the EQ-5D (see Szende et al. 2007), and this is reflected in the way questionnaire respondents' profile data is summed. These EQ-5D values—which are sometimes referred to in the literature as the EQ-5D Index, or quality of life weights or utilities—are constructed to lie on a scale anchored by the value 1, full health, and 0, dead. EQ-5D values cannot take a value higher than 1, but values less than 0 are possible for health states considered to be worse than dead.

A full set of values for each possible EQ-5D profile is often called a 'value set'. These values are obtained from stated preference studies, where members of the general public[4] are asked to imagine living in health states described by the EQ-5D descriptive system, and to engage in a series of tasks designed to gauge how good or bad they consider those health states to be. A variety of methods can be used to elicit these preferences and to model them to create weights for the components of

---

[4]By convention, and for normative reasons, the general public's stated preferences are usually argued to be those relevant to constructing these value sets (see, for example, Neumann et al. 2017). Value sets and their use are discussed in more details in Chap. 4.

- We would like to know how good or bad your health is TODAY.

- This scale is numbered from 0 to 100.

- 100 means the <u>best</u> health you can imagine.
  0 means the <u>worst</u> health you can imagine.

- Mark an X on the scale to indicate how your health is TODAY.

- Now, please write the number you marked on the scale in the

  box below.

YOUR HEALTH TODAY =

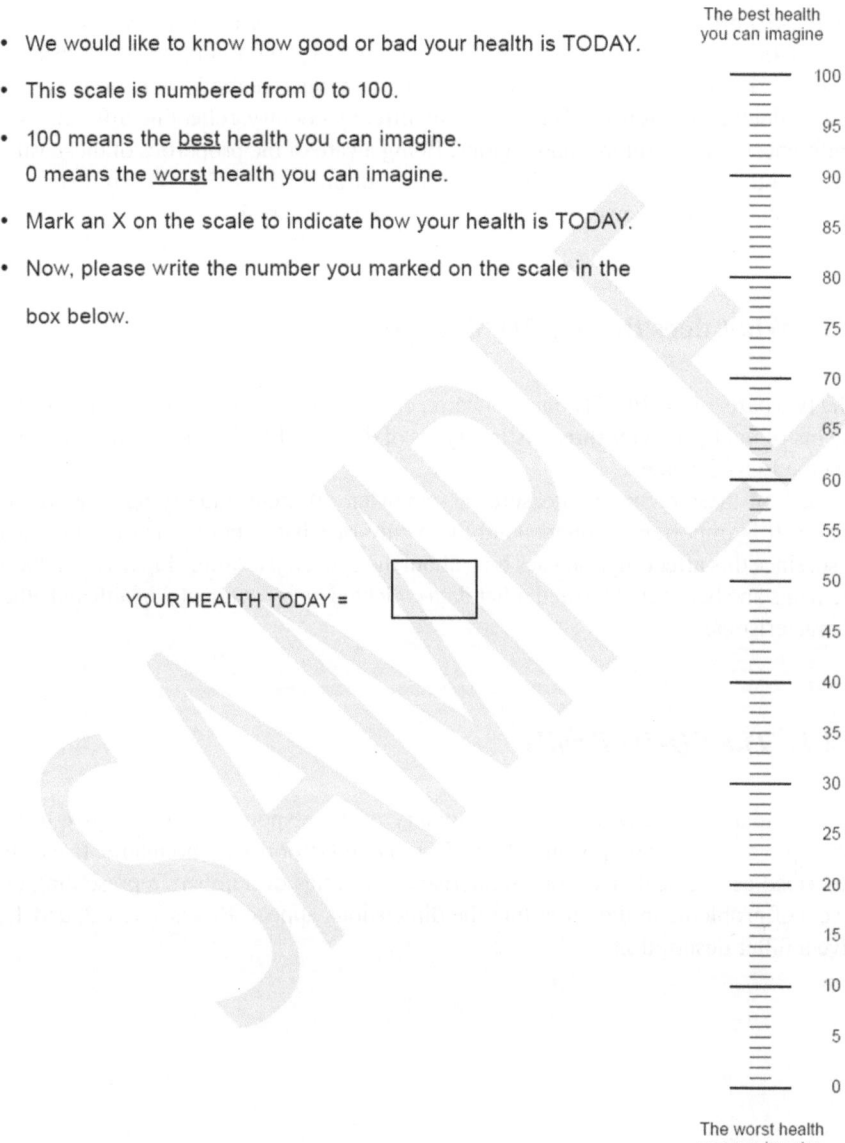

Fig. 1.4 EQ VAS (current EQ-5D-5L and EQ-5D-3L version). *Source* EuroQol Research Foundation. *EQ-5D-5L User Guide, 2019*. Latest version available from: https://euroqol.org/publications/user-guides

the EQ-5D profiles. The resulting 'value sets'—the complete lists of values for each of the 243 profiles described by the EQ-5D-3L and EQ-5D-Y, and for the 3125 states described by the EQ-5D-5L—differ depending on what methods were used to elicit and model the preferences. They may also differ by country, reflecting differences in preferences across cultures and regions. Being aware of the properties of these value sets, and the difference they might make to your analysis of EQ-5D profile data, is important, and we discuss this further below and in Chap. 4.

1.2   What does the EQ-5D Measure?

The two parts of the EQ-5D questionnaire, combined with the value sets, means that the instrument generates three distinct types of data: the EQ-5D profile; the EQ VAS; and the EQ-5D values.

Each of these elements measures a somewhat different underlying construct of health. It is important to understand the nature of what is being measured in each case, since this affects hypotheses both about the expected relationship between these elements and between them and other data collected on respondents' health and other characteristics.

1.2.1   The EQ-5D Profile

A respondent's EQ-5D profile is a summary of the responses that they give to the descriptive system component of the EQ-5D self-report questionnaire. It can be described as five sentences, or summarised as a series of numbers representing the levels of problems in the order that the dimensions appear. Boxes 1.1, 1.2, and 1.3 give a fuller description.

Box 1.1. What are EQ-5D profiles?

A set of responses to the statements given in the descriptive system element of the EQ-5D questionnaire describes a health state or 'profile' as a combination of dimensions and levels within dimensions. For example, a completed questionnaire may be like this:

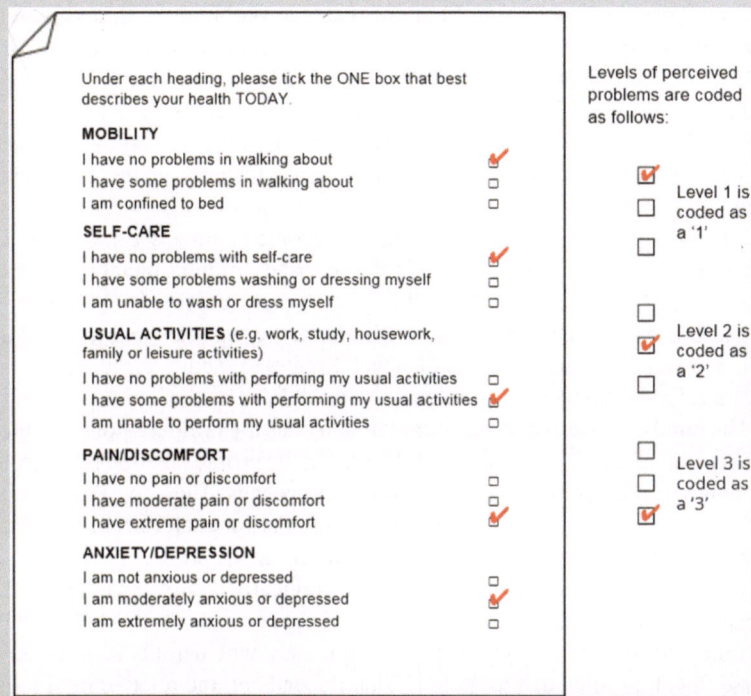

This profile can be described as a series of five sentences. For example, this respondent has:

- No problems in walking about
- No problems with self-care
- Some problems with performing their usual activities
- Extreme pain or discomfort
- Moderate anxiety or depression

In Box 1.2 we describe how these profiles may be more concisely summarised.

Box 1.2. Summarising EQ-5D profiles

A simpler way than using five sentences to summarise a profile is to assign each level a number and describe the profile as a five-number string, representing the level of each dimension in the order in which they appear in the questionnaire. The numbers used are: no problems = 1; some problems = 2; and extreme problems or unable to = 3. So, for example, no problems in any dimension is 11111, some problems in every dimension is 22222, and extreme problems in every dimension is 33333. The profile shown in Box 1.1 is 11232.

EQ-5D-5L profile data can be summarised in the same way. 11111 again means no problem on any of the five dimensions of health and the worst health state is 55555. The profile labels are not directly equivalent between the 3L and the 5L, except for 11111, which means no problems on any dimension. The worst health profiles, 33333 and 55555, describe different underlying health states because the worst level for mobility in the 3L is 'confined to bed' whereas in the 5L it is 'unable to walk about'. Similarly, the 'middle' states, 22222 and 33333, mean different things, as 3L level 2 refers to 'some' problems, but 5L level 3 refers to 'moderate' problems.

The numbers given to levels within dimensions are ordinal—for example, 3 is worse than 2 and 2 is worse than 1. However, the profile labels are categories, not numbers, and do not even have ordinal properties. They do have a limited logical ordering—see Devlin et al. (2010) and Parkin et al. (2010) for further details—and in some cases can be used to compare profiles. For example, profile 11111 is better than profile 11112 (it logically dominates it) and 11112 is better than 11122. But we cannot say anything about *how much* better 11111 is compared to 11112. Moreover, we cannot say whether 11112 is better or worse than a profile such as 11121. That depends on the relative importance attached to some problems with anxiety & depression compared with some problems with pain & discomfort.

Chapter 2 demonstrates how health profiles can be compared to make judgements about whether health has improved, using only the ordinal properties of the levels within profiles. But to compare health profiles such as 11112 and 11121 and to measure the magnitude of the difference between any profiles requires a scoring system that assigns weights to each profile. EQ-5D value sets achieve that, using data from stated preferences studies to convert the profile data into a single, cardinal number. We examine the use of value sets in detail in Chap. 4.

Box 1.3. How many EQ-5D profiles?

For the EQ-5D-3L, there are $3^5 = 243$ possible profiles. There are three groups of profiles that include only two levels (1 and 2, 2 and 3 or 1 and 3), with $2^5 = 32$ profiles (13% of all profiles) in each group. Therefore, for each level there are $3^5–2^5 = 211$ profiles that include at least one of that level. So:

- 32 (13%) do not include a level 3 in any dimension
- 32 (13%) include only level 2 and 3
- 211 (87%) include at least one level 1
- 211 (87%) include at least one level 3

The number of unique profiles described by the EQ-5D-5L is $5^5 = 3125$. There are five groups of profiles that include only four levels, with $4^5 = 1024$ profiles (33% of all profiles) in each group. Therefore, for each level there are $5^5–4^5 = 2101$ profiles that include at least one of that level, $5^5–3^5 = 2882$ that contain at least one of each of two different levels and $5^5–2^5 = 3100$ that contain at least one of each of three different levels. So:

- 1024 (33%) do not include a level 1 in any dimension
- 1024 (33%) do not include a level 5 in any dimension
- 2101 (67%) include at least one level 5
- 2882 (92%) include at least one level 4 or a level 5
- 32 (1%) include only levels 1 and 2
- 32 (1%) include only levels 4 and 5
- 3093 (99%) include levels 1, 3 and 5
- 243 (8%) include only levels 1, 3 and 5.

In practice, not all profiles have an equal probability of being observed. For example, data obtained from the general population often contain a large proportion of profile 11111. In patient data sets, observations are often clustered on a sub-set of profiles relevant to those patients' condition; and some profiles are almost never observed because they contain unusual combinations of levels—for example the EQ-5D-3L profile 33133, in which there are extreme problems with everything except usual activities, where there are no problems.

The profile element of the EQ-5D questionnaire can be categorised as an example of a Health Status Measurement questionnaire, broadly defined (Bowling 2001, 2004). As noted earlier, the EQ-5D is often also described in the literature as measuring HRQoL. However, the concept of quality of life, and which aspects of it are seen as health-related, is often not precisely defined. Because the EQ-5D is a generic instrument, the EQ-5D profile will not capture everything that matters to all people with respect to their health status or HRQoL, and does not claim to do so. That means that, for some diseases and patients, there may be aspects of health that are important which the EQ-5D does not fully reflect, and this may be important to consider in your analysis of the data.

1.2.2 EQ VAS

The EQ VAS can be thought of as showing how patients feel about their own health overall. Their overall score will reflect both the relative importance that they place on the different aspects of their health that are included in the EQ-5D descriptive system and other dimensions of health that are not. The EQ VAS therefore provides information that is complementary to the EQ-5D profile. For example, it is often observed that some people who report no problems in any EQ-5D dimension rate their health as less than 100 on the EQ VAS (for example, see Devlin et al. 2004). Chapter 3 discusses other evidence for this, for example that the average EQ VAS scores decline with age even for those whose profile is 11111. Further, although profiles are systematically related to the EQ VAS scores in regression analyses, they only partially explain them (Feng et al. 2014).

1.2.3 EQ-5D Values

As noted above, EQ-5D values data are produced by applying value sets to summarise the EQ-5D profile data. The nature of these value sets, and their characteristics, are influenced by their principal application, which is in the estimation of quality-adjusted life years (QALYs). It is their use in this context that determines the anchors for the scale of 1 for full health and 0 for dead.[5]

It is important to note that using these value sets to generate EQ-5D values data introduces a source of exogenous variance into the analysis of profile data which can bias statistical inference (Parkin et al. 2010). Each value set places a different weight on the various levels and dimensions of the profile data, reflecting underlying differences in preferences, the methods used to elicit them, or both. This means that whether there are statistically significant differences in the EQ-5D values between, for example, two arms of a clinical trial, or between two regions in a national health survey, may depend on which value set is used, and the relative importance it puts on the different types of health problems and improvements in them.

More generally, there is *no* neutral way to summarise the data from the EQ-5D profile into a single number. This is not an issue that is only relevant to the EQ-5D instruments: these same points are relevant to the scoring and weighting systems used in *all* generic or condition specific PROs. Any method of combining responses to multiple questions must entail some weight being placed on each question. Even if preference-based weights were not used, and the dimensions of a PRO were equally weighted, that would imply a strong value judgement about the relative importance of various kinds of health problems that may or may not reflect the views of the people who self-reported their health on that PRO. Analysts should be aware of this, and check for the sensitivity of results to the choice of value set.

---

[5]The convention of anchoring at dead = 0 is very widely accepted, but could be debated—see Sampson et al. (2019).

1.2.4   Which Aspect of the Information Provided by the EQ-5D Should be the Primary Focus of My Analysis?

When considering which element of the EQ-5D data should be the primary focus of analysis, and what methods of analysis should be used, users should be guided by the *purpose* of collecting EQ-5D data and how the results will be used. Table 1.1 provides an overview of the main contexts in which EQ-5D data are collected, and implications regarding the analysis of the resulting data.

There are advantages in being able to summarise and represent a health profile by a single number like the EQ-5D values—for example, it simplifies statistical analysis. However, as we have already emphasised, there is no neutral set of weights that can be used for that purpose: they all embody judgements about what is meant by importance and the appropriate source of information for judging importance. It is therefore not possible to offer generalised guidance about which set of weights should be used if the sole purpose is to summarise profile data for descriptive or inferential statistical analysis. Users should consider the wider purpose for which the summary will be used. If the purpose is simply to provide descriptive information, then it may be better not to use EQ-5D values, but to focus analysis on the profile data themselves (see Chap. 2). This may also be preferable because the EQ-5D value provides less detailed information than the EQ-5D profile it is summarising. Focussing on the EQ-5D values may obscure the underlying information on the type and severity of problems affecting patients that the profile data provide (for example, see Gutacker et al. 2013).

Further, in some cases where a single number is required to represent health, for example, in the generation of population norms (Kind et al. 1999), it may be more appropriate to focus on the EQ VAS data provided by patients or populations, rather than applying the EQ-5D value sets to their profile data.

Economic Evaluation

Where the economic evaluation of treatment is the main goal of analysis, this has implications for the analysis of EQ-5D data. A key requirement for a health measure to use in cost effectiveness analysis is that it should provide an unambiguous measure of effectiveness. That is, higher EQ values should represent a better state of health and the same differences between EQ values should have the same level of importance. For example, the difference between 0.87 and 0.91 should represent the same degree of change as between 0.22 and 0.26. However, there is arguably a further requirement if the measure of effectiveness is to be based on economics principles, such as those embodied in cost utility analysis—essentially, that the weights need to represent 'values.' Just as costs represent the total value of resources used, that is the volume of each type of resource weighted by their individual value, effectiveness in the context of economic evaluation should represent the value of health output, that is the amount of health generated weighted by its value.

Table 1.1 Example of types of studies and some considerations for analysis

Types of studies or health care contexts in which EQ-5D data are collected	What questions are being asked?	What are the implications for data analysis?
Clinical trials	Is this technology effective and cost-effective relative to the comparator in the sample of patients included in this trial?	EQ-5D values are required for estimation of QALY gains. The EQ-5D profile and EQ VAS can provide additional evidence on relative effectiveness. Cluster analysis can be used to identify responder/non-responder groups
Observational studies of patient populations	The focus of these studies varies but could include: how does self-reported health change through time in a given patient group? How do patients' health compare to the general public? What evidence is there of response to treatment?	Descriptive analysis of EQ-5D profile and EQ VAS at each observation and analysis of changes between repeated observations. EQ-5D values will be required if estimation of QALYs is a goal. Cluster analysis can be used to identify responder/non-responder groups
Population health surveys	How does the health of a population compare with that of others? What is the burden of ill health?	Comparisons of EQ-5D profile and EQ VAS between sub-populations. EQ-5D values can provide a means of summarising profile data as a single number (although there are caveats about the use of values in this context, as we note in the following paragraphs)
Routine data collection in the health care system ('PROMs programmes')	How much variation is there between providers in improving patient health? How do patients' health and health improvements compare between different conditions and treatments? How does the cost effectiveness of different procedures compare?	Comparisons of profile and EQ VAS. EQ-5D values can be used as a way of summarising profile data as a single number, although caution is required (see p. 12) EQ-5D values are relevant where QALY estimation is required
Shared decision making between a patient and their doctor	What problems is this patient reporting? How difficult do they find these problems overall? How should this effect choice of treatment?	The individual patient's profile and EQ VAS are the focus. These may be benchmarked against evidence from other patients

There is ongoing debate over the extent to which the commonly-used stated preferences methods used adequately reflect underlying notions of 'value', and about the adequacy of QALYs as a measure of societal benefit from treating ill health. However, there appears to be general acceptance (for example, among Health Technology Appraisal bodies, like the National Health Care Institute (Zorginstituut) in The Netherlands, and the United Kingdom's National Institute for Health and Care Excellence) that value sets available for EQ-5D instruments, based on the preferences of adult members of the general public, are usually appropriate for use in cost effectiveness analysis (NICE 2013; Zorginstituut Nederland 2016; Neumann et al. 2017).

Further detail on EQ-5D values, including which value set to use, and the analysis of EQ-5D values data, is provided in Chap. 4.

1.3 EQ-5D Data Collection and Data Handling

Where EQ-5D data are captured electronically, manual data entry is not required. However, in many cases, EQ-5D questionnaires are still completed in paper format. Where this is the case, data will need to be coded and entered manually. As this process is subject to human error, best practice for EQ-5D questionnaires is the same as any other self-completed paper questionnaire and entails double entry—that is, data being entered twice, and files compared for anomalies, which are then checked against the hardcopy.

Coding and data entry for the descriptive system are relatively straightforward. It is recommended that levels are coded as 1, 2 and 3 (for the EQ-5D-3L) and 1, 2, 3, 4 and 5 (for the EQ-5D-5L) in each dimension, to enable easy generation of the conventional 5-number profile label. Missing data need to be flagged as do any unusual responses, for example if more than one level is ticked on a dimension, although the latter are relatively rare.

EQ VAS data collected electronically are also very straightforward. However, the paper format of the original and current versions of the EQ VAS used in the EQ-5D-3L and EQ-5D-5L (see Figs. 1.4 and 1.5) and the current version of the EQ-5D-Y (see Fig. 1.6) require respondents to draw a line or mark a cross on the VAS to record their response. The resulting data can require a considerable degree of interpretation in coding responses. For example, Feng et al. (2014) noted, from qualitative analysis of a sub-sample of English National Health Service (NHS) PROMs data, a number of common response types with respect to the EQ VAS data (see Table 1.2).

Whereas a type 1 response in Table 1.2 is the only response which strictly complies with the EQ VAS instructions, Feng et al. (2014) argue that types 2 and 3 also provide unambiguous responses that can be captured accurately and reflect the same meaning to the score intended by respondents. Together, types 1–3 covered 88% respondents in the data presented in Table 1.2. Other types, including missing and ambiguous responses (types 5 and 6) require separate codes to flag these issues in analysis. Similar issues may exist with EQ VAS data from the EQ-5D-Y.

To help people say how good or bad a health state is, we have drawn a scale (rather like a thermometer) on which the best state you can imagine is marked **100** and the worst state you can imagine is marked **0**.

We would like you to indicate on this scale how good or bad your own health is today, in your opinion. Please do this by drawing a line from the box below to whichever point on the scale indicates how good or bad your health state is today.

Your own health state today

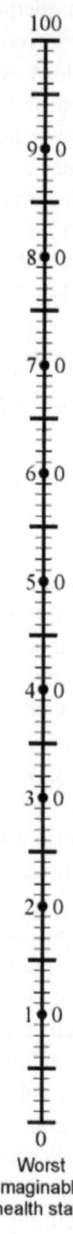

Best
imaginable
health state

100

90

80

70

60

50

40

30

20

10

0

Worst
imaginable
health state

Fig. 1.5 EQ VAS (Original EQ-5D-3L version). *Source* EuroQol Research Foundation. *EQ-5D-3L User Guide, 2015*. Latest version available from: https://euroqol.org/publications/user-guides

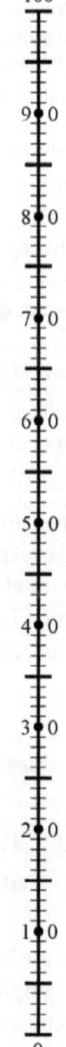

The best health
you can imagine

How good is your health TODAY

- We would like to know how good or bad your health is
  TODAY.
- This line is numbered from 0 to 100.
- 100 means the <u>best</u> health you can imagine.
  0 means the <u>worst</u> health you can imagine.
- Please mark an X on the line that shows how good or bad
  your health is TODAY.

Fig. 1.6 EQ VAS (EQ-5D-Y version). *Source* EuroQol Research Foundation. *EQ-5D-Y User Guide, 2014*. Latest version available from: https://euroqol.org/publications/user-guides

Table 1.2 Types of responses to the original EQ-5D-3L EQ VAS

	EQ VAS response type, from most to least frequent	% responses
1	Drew a line from the box towards the EQ VAS, sometimes touching or crossing it. This is the way that the EuroQol Group intends the EQ VAS to be completed	45
2	Indicated precisely a horizontal level on the VAS, but did not draw a line to it. For example, ticks, crosses, lines, arrows, asterisks on or beside the VAS, or a tightly drawn circle around a specific number or tick mark	32
3	Drew a vertical line extending from 0 up to a point parallel with a point on the VAS	11
4	Missing	8
5	Drew a vertical line parallel to the VAS, but not extending from 0, or circled an area of the VAS. This indicated a range rather than a single point	4
6	Gave an unclear response. For example, multiple markings on the VAS or vertical lines drawn from 100 downwards	1

Source Feng et al. (2014). Response types have been combined across both pre-and post-surgery responses and re-ordered by frequency

The current format of the EQ VAS in the EQ-5D-5L and EQ-5D-3L (see Fig. 1.4) entails respondents both noting a number in the box and marking a cross on the scale. In electronic data capture, the two are identical. In paper completion, there is potential for the two responses to differ, and best practice would suggest capturing both and reporting any such discrepancies.

1.4   Before Starting Your Analysis

1.4.1   Treatment of Missing Data—What to Do, What Not to Do

There are broadly two types of missing EQ-5D data. Data can be missing altogether—for example, where an elective surgery patient in the English NHS fails to complete and return their post-surgery PROMs questionnaire. Or data can be missing in part—for example, where the patient completes an EQ-5D questionnaire, but provides incomplete profile data, or does not complete the EQ VAS.

General guidelines (i.e. relating to PRO data, rather than specifically the EQ-5D) often indicate that a substantial amount of missing data can compromise the validity of analysis—but what constitutes 'substantial' is a matter of opinion. For example, based on the German Institute for Quality and Efficiency in Health Care (Institut für Qualität und Wirtschaftlichkeit im Gesundheitswesen) standard approach, data from at least 70% of patients at both baseline and one follow up visit are needed to consider analysis of that data valid for its purposes. However, 'percent missing' is not defined consistently across the literature and different definitions on how to estimate the amount of missing data may lead to different practices and results (Coens et al. 2020). Further, even where there are high rates of missing data, analysis of available data may still yield insights into the sub-group who did respond, even if results cannot be generalised to non-responders. In short, there are no hard and fast rules. However, it is important for analysts to report missing data, and to be mindful of potential limitations arising from loss of generalisability.

In general, you should provide data descriptions, state the assumptions underlying the handling of the missing EQ-5D data, and conduct sensitivity analyses to the selected assumption. Included in the data description should be the amount of missing data, missing data patterns, and the association between missing data and observed data, for example respondents' age, gender and any previously observed EQ-5D data for that respondent (Faria et al. 2014).

Analytical methods used for missing data in general are applicable to the EQ-5D; users are advised to consult a statistical text for details. Essentially, it is necessary to consider the assumed form that missingness takes for the data—Missing Completely At Random (MCAR), Missing At Random (MAR) or Missing Not At Random (MNAR) (Little and Rubin 1987)—and to select a method for dealing with this appropriate to that form.

If MCAR, where a respondent's missing data are not related to that person's socio-demographic or other characteristics, analysis can assume that the missing data follow the same patterns as the non-missing data.

If MAR, where a respondent's missing data is related to their observed characteristics, but not any unobserved characteristics, analysis can assume that we have a random sample of respondents with those characteristics and make inferences from that sample about the data that are missing. Multiple Imputation (MI) has been increasingly used in recent years for EQ-5D data with MAR (Ratcliffe et al. 2005; Kaambwa et al. 2012; Simons et al. 2015).

If MNAR, where a respondent's data are missing because of their characteristics, we do not have random samples of people with different characteristics and require more complex analytical methods to deal with resulting selection bias. The Heckman selection model has been applied to EQ-5D values data that are assumed to be MNAR (Kaambwa et al. 2012).

Recent guidance suggests that data analysts should evaluate the sensitivity of the analysis to the MAR assumption using methods such as the weighting or pattern mixture approaches (Faria et al. 2014; Simons et al. 2015). In particular the evaluation should examine how the results might change when a MNAR assumption is made to the missing EQ-5D data.

There are two missing data issues specific to EQ-5D data. First, there is the issue of what should be done where the user wishes to analyse profiles and some but not all of the profile items are missing. Bad practice includes substituting for a respondent's missing profile items an average derived from their non-missing items and substituting an average derived from the non-missing items in the sample as a whole. It might be possible to use MI in this context, but there are currently no examples on which to base guidance. Conservative guidance is therefore to treat as missing any profiles based on missing profile items.

The second is where some or all of the profile items are missing, and the user wishes to analyse EQ-5D values. For this, MI may be an appropriate method if the data are assumed MAR, but an issue is whether this should be applied to profile items, from which an EQ-5D value is calculated, or to EQ-5D values directly (Faria et al. 2014). In practice, the decision depends on the observed missing data pattern and the sample size available for analysis (Simons et al. 2015).

1.4.2 Planning Your Analysis

A systematic review of the use of PROs in oncology conducted by the Setting International Standards in Analyzing Patient-Reported Outcomes and Quality of Life Endpoints Data (SISAQOL) Consortium (Pe et al. 2018) showed a widespread lack of clearly-specified a priori research hypotheses and a link with the design and statistical methods to be employed. New guidelines for protocol development (for example SPIRIT-PRO) and reporting of PROs (for example CONSORT-PRO[6]—see Calvert et al. 2013) also recognise this to be a common issue in PRO studies generally.

Before beginning analysis of EQ-5D data, you should therefore consider what questions you want to answer with your data. What are your hypotheses about, for example, how a treatment arm is expected to behave relative to a reference arm in a clinical trial? What assumptions underpin these hypotheses, for example what is your rationale and what evidence has informed that? This, in turn, should inform the statistical analysis plan (SAP) developed prior to analysis. Note that the content of SAPs will vary depending on the study type and study aims.

1.5 Guide to the Rest of this Book

In the remainder of this book, we explain in detail how each element of the data generated from using EQ-5D instruments—the profile data, EQ VAS and EQ values — can be analysed. We provide both a basic introduction to analysis in each case, assuming no prior knowledge of analysis of EQ-5D data, as well as introducing more advanced topics relating to analysis of EQ-5D data.

---

[6]CONSORT: Consolidated Standards Of Reporting Trials.

References

Appleby J, Devlin N, Parkin D (2015) Using patient reported outcomes to improve health care. Wiley. ISBN: 978-1-118-94860-6

Bowling A (2001) Measuring disease: a review of disease specific quality of life measurement scales, 2nd edn. Open University Press

Bowling A (2004) Measuring health: a review of quality of life measurement scales. McGraw-Hill

Bren L (2006) The Importance of Patient-Reported Outcomes ... It's All About the Patients. FDA Consum 40(6):26–32

Calvert M et al (2018) Guidelines for inclusion of patient-reported outcomes in clinical trial protocols: the SPIRIT-PRO extension. JAMA 6; 319(5):483–494

Calvert M, Blazeby J, Altman DG et al (2013) Reporting of patient reported outcomes in randomised trials. J Am Med Assoc 309(8):814–822

Coens C, Pe M, Dueck AC, Sloan J et al (2020) International standards for the analysis of quality-of-life and patient-reported outcome endpoints in cancer randomised controlled trials: recommendations of the SISAQOL Consortium. Lancet Oncol 21(2):e83–e96

Devlin N, Brooks R (2017) EQ-5D and the EuroQol Group: past, present, future. Appl Health Econ Health Policy 15(2):127–137

Devlin N, Hansen P, Selai C (2004) Understanding health state valuations: a qualitative analysis of respondents' comments. Qual Life Res 13(7):1265–1277

Devlin NJ, Parkin D, Browne J (2010) Patient-reported outcome measures in the NHS: new methods for analysing and reporting EQ-5D data. Health Econ 19(8):886–905

European Medicines Agency (2006) Reflection paper on the regulatory guidance for the use of health related quality of life (HRQL) measures in the evaluation of medicinal products. EMA: Committee for medicinal products in human use. https://www.ema.europa.eu/documents/sci entific-guideline/reflection-paper-regulatory-guidance-use-healthrelated-quality-life-hrql-mea sures-evaluation_en.pdf. Accessed 18 Dec 2018

Faria R, Gomes M, Epstein D, White IR (2014) A guide to handling missing data in cost-effectiveness analysis conducted within randomised controlled trials. Pharmacoeconomics 32(12):1157–1170

FDA (2009) Guidance for industry patient-reported outcome measures: use in medical product development to support labeling claims. https://www.fda.gov/downloads/drugs/guidances/ucm 193282.pdf. Accessed 18 Dec 2018

Feng Y, Parkin D, Devlin N (2014) Assessing the performance of the EQ VAS in the NHS PROMS programme. Qual Life Res 23(3):977–989

Gutacker N, Bojke C, Daidone S, Devlin N, Street A (2013) Hospital variation in patient-reported outcome at the level of EQ-5D dimensions: evidence from England. Med Decis Making 33(6):804–818

Herdman M, Gudex C, Lloyd A, Janssen M, Kind P, Parkin D, Bonsel G, Badia X (2011) Development and preliminary testing of the new five-level version of EQ-5D (EQ-5D-5L). Qual Life Res 20(10):1727–1736

Kaambwa B, Bryan S, Billingham L (2012) Do the methods used to analyse missing data really matter? An examination of data from an observational study of Intermediate Care patients. BMC Res Notes 5:330

Kind P, Hardman H, Macran S (1999) UK population norms for EQ-5D. Working Papers 172 Centre for Health Economics, University of York

Little RJA, Rubin DB (1987) Statistical analysis with missing data. Wiley, New York

Matza LS, Patrick D, Riley AW et al (2013) Pediatric patient-reported outcome instruments for research to support medical product labeling: report of the ISPOR PRO good research practices for the assessment of children and adolescents task force. Value Health 16:461–479

Morris S, Devlin N, Parkin D, Spencer A (2012) Economic analysis in health care, 2nd edn. Wiley

Neumann PJ, Sanders GD, Russell LB, Siegel JE, Ganiats TG (2017) Cost effectiveness in health and medicine, 2nd edn. Oxford University Press

NICE (2013) Guide to the methods of technology appraisal. https://www.nice.org.uk/process/pmg9/ chapter/foreword. Accessed 18 Dec 2018

Parkin D, Rice N, Devlin N (2010) Statistical analysis of EQ-5D profiles: does the use of value sets bias inference? Med Decis Making 30(5):556–565

Patrick DL, Erickson P (1993) Health status and health policy: quality of life in health care evaluation and resource allocation. Oxford University Press, New York

Pe M, Dorme L, Coens C, Basch E, Calvert M, Campbell A, Cleeland C, Cocks K, Collette L, Dirven L, Dueck AC, Devlin N, Flechtner HH, Gotay C, Griebsch I, Groenvold M, King M, Koller M, Malone DC, Martinelli F, Mitchell SA, Musoro JZ, Oliver K, Piault-Louis E, Piccart M, Pimentel FL, Quinten C, Reijneveld JC, Sloan J, Velikova G, Bottomley A (2018) Setting international standards in analyzing patient-reported outcomes and quality of life endpoints data consortium (SISAQOL). Lancet Oncol 19(9):e459–e469

Ratcliffe J, Young T, Longworth L, Buxton M (2005) An assessment of the impact of informative dropout and nonresponse in measuring health-related quality of life using the EuroQol (EQ-5D) descriptive system. Value Health 8(1):53–58

Sampson C, Parkin D, Devlin N (2019) Drop dead: is anchoring at 'dead' a theoretical requirement in health state valuation? Paper presented to the 35th scientific plenary meeting of the EuroQol Group, Barcelona, Spain

Simons CL, Rivero-Arias O, Yu LM, Simon J (2015) Multiple imputation to deal with missing EQ-5D-3L data: should we impute individual domains or the actual index? Qual Life Res 24(4):805–815

Szende A, Oppe M, Devlin N (2007) EQ-5D value sets: inventory, comparative review and user guide. Springer

Wille N, Badia X, Bonsel G et al (2010) Development of the EQ-5D-Y: a child-friendly version of the EQ-5D. Qual Life Res 19(6):875–886

Zbrozek A, Hebert J, Gogates G et al (2013) Validation of electronic systems to collect patient-reported outcome (PRO) data—recommendations for clinical trial teams: report of the ISPOR ePRO systems validation good research practices task force. Value Health 16:480–489

Zorginstituut Nederland (2016) Guideline for economic evaluation in health care. https://tools. ispor.org/PEguidelines/source/Netherlands_Guideline_for_economic_evaluations_in_health care.pdf. Accessed 3 July 2019

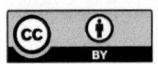

Chapter 2
Analysis of EQ-5D Profiles

The aims of this chapter are

- to demonstrate a variety of analyses that can be performed on the profile data generated from the EQ-5D instruments: EQ-5D-3L, EQ-5D-5L and EQ-5D-Y;
- to explain methods that can be used to describe EQ-5D profile data in cross-sectional (collected at a single point in time) and longitudinal (describing changes over time) designs; and
- to consider the advantages and limitations of each method, and outline in which decision contexts insights from them might be useful.

Profile data form the cornerstone of analyses of EQ-5D data and, in many cases, are likely to be the primary focus of interest. In this chapter, we provide an overview of methods that can be used to describe the profile data from respondents at a given point in time, and to describe the changes in profiles between different points in time.

Even when the ultimate goal of analysis is to generate EQ-5D values and to estimate quality-adjusted life years (QALYs), analysis of profile data provides important insights and should always be the starting point for analysts. For example, summarising EQ-5D patient data simply as values obscures the underlying information about which aspects of their health have been most affected by their condition, or improved by treatment. To know about that, you need to look at the data that respondents have given you: the boxes they ticked on an EQ-5D questionnaire.

The methods presented here need not be treated as alternatives, but rather as complementary. Although they are illustrated using EQ-5D data, and in some cases developed specifically for the analysis of EQ-5D profile data, these same methods could just as readily be applied to other generic or condition specific health status or patient reported outcome (PRO) measures.

It should be noted that we do not cover inferential statistics, either hypothesis testing or estimation, as this book is not intended as a statistical primer and we assume that readers will be able to apply appropriate inference procedures where required. For example, we describe contingency tables, to which measures of association such as a $\chi 2$ test could be applied.

© The Author(s) 2020
N. Devlin et al., *Methods for Analysing and Reporting EQ-5D Data*,
https://doi.org/10.1007/978-3-030-47622-9_2

2.1   Cross-Sectional Analysis: Describing Health at a Point in Time by Dimension and Level

Exploratory data analysis (EDA) of EQ-5D data, including the use of simple descriptive statistics, is undervalued, and often underreported in papers that contain more complex econometric and psychometric analyses. This is bad practice and wasteful of information, because EDA not only generates information that helps in interpreting more complex analyses, but also generates information about health within populations and about the properties of the EQ-5D which is valuable in itself.

Describing health at the most detailed level possible for the EQ-5D can be done very simply, by reporting the number and percentage of patients reporting each level of problem on each dimension of the EQ-5D. An example of this is shown in Table 2.1, which shows EQ-5D-3L data provided by patients before and after hip surgery, using data from a pilot study for the Patient Reported Outcome Measures (PROMs) programme in the English National Health Service (NHS) (Devlin et al. 2010).

This very simple table provides some important information. For example, before hip surgery, 420 of these patients (95.7% of the sample) reported a level 2 problem on mobility, but none reported a level 3 problem. The reason is that Level 3 on the EQ-5D-3L mobility dimension is 'confined to bed'—and even patients with very poor mobility because of hip problems aren't confined to bed. That is a problem with the EQ-5D-3L—as has been pointed out previously (Oppe et al. 2011). This issue has been corrected in the EQ-5D-5L (Herdman et al. 2011), where the most severe problem with mobility is 'unable to walk about', and is an important advantage of the 5L over the 3L (Janssen et al. 2018).

The information on the types of problems experienced by a sample of patients at any given point in time can be simplified still further by collapsing levels together, to create just two categories: the number and percentage of patients reporting no problems (level 1), and the number reporting any level of problems (levels 2 and 3 for the 3L, and levels 2, 3, 4 and 5 for the 5L). This can also be seen in Table 2.1. For example, before surgery, mobility problems are common in these patients, as might be expected: only 4.3% of these patients had no problems with mobility. Of the 95.7% of patients who reported having at least some problem on mobility before surgery, all reported a level 2, as noted above. However, problems on other dimensions are just as prevalent: 99.8% of patients reported at least some problem with pain and discomfort, and 96.6% at least some problem with usual activities. Over 40% of these patients also reported problems with anxiety and depression—something that might be missed by condition specific instruments focused on mobility and function-related issues specific to hips, such as the Oxford Hip Score.

Examining the profile data by each dimension and level in this manner is a good starting point to understanding the nature of the health problems reported in the data you have collected. However, there are limitations to this way of reporting the data. Because the focus is on the frequency of observations in each level *within* each dimension, it doesn't tell us how these problems combine in the people reporting

Table 2.1 Frequency of levels by dimension of 'some problems', before and after elective hip surgery in the English NHS

Level	Mobility		Self-care		Usual activities		Pain and discomfort		Anxiety and depression	
	Pre-op	Post-op	Pre-op	Post-op	Pre-op	Post-op	Pre-op	Post-op	Pre-op	Post-op
1	19 (4.3%)	239 (54.4%)	168 (38.6%)	319 (73.3%)	15 (3.4%)	199 (45.6%)	1 (0.2%)	219 (50.5%)	240 (55.5%)	349 (80.8%)
2	420 (95.7%)	200 (45.6%)	264 (60.7%)	115 (26.4%)	347 (79.6%)	221 (50.7%)	240 (55.3%)	200 (46.1%)	183 (42.4%)	74 (17.1%)
3	0 (0%)	0 (0%)	3 (0.7%)	1 (0.2%)	74 (17.0%)	16 (3.7%)	193 (44.5%)	15 (3.4%)	9 (2.1%)	9 (2.1%)
Total[a]	439 (100%)	439 (100%)	435 (100%)	435 (100%)	436 (100%)	436 (100%)	434 (100%)	434 (100%)	432 (100%)	432 (100%)
Number reporting some problems[b]	420 (95.7%)	200 (45.6%)	267 (61.4%)	116 (26.6%)	421 (96.6%)	237 (54.4%)	433 (99.8%)	215 (49.5%)	192 (44.5%)	83 (19.2%)
Change in numbers reporting problems	−220		−151		−184		−218		−109	
% change in numbers reporting problems	−52%		−57%		−44%		−53%		−57%	
Rank of dimensions in terms of % changes	3		1		4		2		1	

[a]Results are for those who responded to both the pre- and the post-operative EQ-5D. 84% of respondents to the pre-operative EQ-5D also responded to the post-operative EQ-5D
[b]'Some problems' = levels 2 + 3
Source Devlin et al. (2010)

them. For example, are the people who report a level 3 on Anxiety and Depression also the same people who report a level 3 on Usual Activities? For this reason, it is also important to examine the way that observed levels of problems on each dimension combine into EQ-5D profiles, which is covered in Sect. 2.3.

2.2   Longitudinal Analysis: Describing Changes in Health Between Two Time Points by Dimension and Level

In addition to describing health states at any one point in time, if you have collected EQ-5D profile data at more than one time point, you are likely also to be interested in describing the changes between them—for example, before and after surgery, or between various time points in a clinical trial, compared to baseline. This too can be done at the level of the EQ-5D dimensions, as is also shown in Table 2.1.

'Eyeballing' the differences in numbers and percentages of patients in each of the levels tells us about the nature of the changes in health that resulted from surgery. For example, the results in Table 2.1 show there were quite striking improvements in patients' Anxiety and Depression, Self-care and Pain and Discomfort—not just Mobility. And because of the issue with level 3 Mobility noted above, whereby the worst level of problem these patients were likely to report on mobility was level 2, the only improvements to mobility that were possible as a result of hip replacement surgery were from 'some' to 'no' problems. This issue with the use of the EQ-5D-3L to measure health outcomes from hip surgery would not have been apparent if these patients' data had been analysed just in terms of EQ-5D values.

It can however be difficult readily to get an overall picture of improvements, even for these relatively simple EQ-5D-3L data. As with the analysis of cross-sectional data, this does not summarise the extent of improvement across dimensions. As noted in Sect. 2.1, one way of handling this is to collapse the levels into just two categories: no problems and some problems. The shift between these two categories provides a simpler way of capturing change. The change in health between time points, reported in this manner, provides a way of summarising the overall extent to which patients go from any level of problem to no problem within each dimension. This may be useful in some contexts, but it has some limitations as an indicator of improvement because of the loss of information caused by aggregation of levels. It doesn't capture improvements other than shifts to no problem, so other improvements that may be of value to patients, for example from extreme to moderate problems, are not captured. That means, that if applied to the EQ-5D-5L, the advantages of its more refined descriptive system will be lost.

2.3 Cross-Sectional Analysis: Describing Health at a Point in Time Using Profiles

While describing the number and percentage of observed levels within each dimension (as in Table 2.1) gives very useful information dimension-by-dimension, it does not tell you anything about the way these problems are *combined* in the health states reported by patients.

One of the most simple and instructive things you can do with an EQ-5D profile data set is to report the cumulative frequency of these profiles. This will reveal the extent to which your observations are evenly distributed over many profiles, or instead concentrated on a relatively small number of health profiles.

The results can sometimes be quite surprising. For example, in Table 2.2 we show the cumulative frequency of self-reported EQ-5D-3L profiles reported by 7294 respondents in the 2012 Health Survey for England. In this example, the great majority of respondents self-reported their health using only a small number of profiles. The top three most frequently reported profiles represented almost three quarters of the respondents.

In contrast, Table 2.3 shows the cumulative frequency of profiles reported by 996 respondents from the general public in the EQ-5D-5L value set study for England for their self-reported health on the EQ-5D-5L. This shows, in comparison to Table 2.2, a larger number of unique health states observed in this data set, and the observations are less concentrated on a small number of states. A large proportion of observations are accounted for by profile 11111 (no problems on any dimension) in both data sets, which is not surprising given that both samples comprise members of the general public, many of whom would not regard themselves as ill. But in general, this 'ceiling effect' is somewhat less in the EQ-5D-5L data (Devlin et al. 2018). Obviously, the

Table 2.2 Prevalence of the 10 most frequently observed self-reported health states and frequency of reporting of the worst possible health state in EQ-5D-3L

Health states	Frequency (%)	Cumulative frequency (%)
11111	4096 (56.2)	56.2
11121	855 (11.7)	67.9
11112	496 (6.8)	74.7
11122	241 (3.3)	78.0
21221	224 (3.1)	81.0
21121	222 (3.0)	84.1
21222	138 (1.9)	86.0
11221	103 (1.4)	87.4
11222	67 (0.9)	88.3
22221	64 (0.9)	89.2
...		
33333	4 (0.1)	100

Source Feng et al. (2015)

Table 2.3 Prevalence of the 10 most frequently observed self-reported health states and frequency of reporting of the worst possible health states in EQ-5D-5L

Health States	Frequency (%)	Cumulative Frequency in (%)
EQ-5D-5L		
11111	474 (47.6)	47.6
11121	93 (9.3)	56.9
11112	46 (4.6)	61.6
11131	22 (2.2)	63.8
21121	21 (2.1)	65.9
11122	21 (2.1)	68.0
21221	19 (1.9)	69.9
11123	13 (1.3)	71.2
21111	11 (1.1)	72.3
11221	11 (1.1)	73.4
...		
55555	0 (0.0)	100

Source Feng et al. (2015)

states observed and their cumulative frequency will differ from data set to data set, but in general the EQ-5D-5L yields less concentrated data, reflecting the advantages of the larger number of response options.

Understanding these patterns of observations in your data is important for three reasons:

(i)   The way self-reported health problems are combined may be useful, as a complement to clinical information, for understanding and planning for patients' treatment needs.

(ii) The combination of problems into health profiles determines the distribution of EQ-5D values data. For example, Parkin et al. (2016) show that the clustering of observations on particular EQ-5D-3L profiles contributes to the unusual 'two group' distribution that is often seen in EQ-5D-3L values data.

(iii) The characteristics of the distribution of problems at baseline may have important implications for the potential for and nature of health improvements that can be observed at later time points.

Looking at the cumulative frequency is a simple and effective way of getting an insight into the distribution of health profiles in a data set. However, a limitation is that it does not provide a summary statistic that allows us readily to (a) describe how good or bad the health states are, or (b) the extent to which the observations cluster on just a few health states, or are evenly spread out over the available heath states described by the descriptive system. Having a summary statistic to characterise the degree to which there is clustering or dispersion of observed health states is useful, especially if one wanted to compare this characteristic, for example to find out whether there are changes in the distribution of profile data from a group of patients observed at different time points, or between EQ-5D profile data from patients with different conditions.

2.4   Longitudinal Analysis: Describing Changes in Health Between Two Time Points Using Profiles

Descriptive analyses of profile data such as Table 2.1 can be very useful, but they contain a lot of information and sometimes an overall summary is required. One way of summarising profile data is to generate a single number for each profile using weights, for example using value sets. However, as noted in Chap. 1, this introduces possible problems of information loss and bias. The good news is that there are ways of summarising changes in EQ-5D health status without using value sets, just using the data that respondents have given you.

2.4.1   The Paretian Classification of Health Change (PCHC)

Devlin et al. (2010) introduced a way of summarising changes in profile data called the Paretian Classification of Health Change (PCHC). The approach is based on the principles of a Pareto improvement in Welfare Economics, drawing an analogy with the challenge of summing up changes in utility of different individuals, where utility can be measured only in ordinal terms. The idea is simple: an EQ-5D health state is deemed to be 'better' than another if it is better on at least one dimension and is no worse on any other dimension. And an EQ-5D health state is deemed to be 'worse' than another if it is worse in at least one dimension and is no better in any other dimension. Using that principle to compare a person's EQ-5D health states between any two time-points, there are only four possibilities:

(i)   Their health state is better
(ii)   Their heath state is worse
(iii) Their health state is the same
(iv) The changes in health are 'mixed': better in at least one dimension, but worse in at least one other.

Applying this to the English NHS PROMs pilot hip replacement data, we found that under 5% had no change, 82% had improved health, under 5% had worse health, and under 10% had a 'mixed' change (Devlin et al. 2010). In other words, this simple analysis provides a very clear summary of what is happening to patients' health because of hip surgery—without relying on value sets. It also highlighted important differences in the benefits from hip surgery, compared with the other types of elective surgery analysed in the English NHS PROMs pilot, shown in Tables 2.4 and 2.5. Looking at Table 2.4, hip replacement operations were by far the best in terms of success in reducing the number of patients who had problems, with knee

Table 2.4 Changes in health for five surgical procedures according to the PCHC

	Hip	Knee	Hernia	Veins	Cataract
No change	21 (4.7%)	45 (10.0%)	127 (29.5%)	72 (27.1%)	335 (47.1%)
Improve	356 (82.0%)	329 (73.3%)	203 (47.2%)	148 (55.6%)	149 (21.0%)
Worsen	18 (4.2%)	34 (7.6%)	71 (16.5%)	34 (12.8%)	188 (26.4%)
Mixed change	39 (9.0%)	41 (9.1%)	29 (6.7%)	12 (4.5%)	39 (5.5%)
Total	434	449	430	266	711

Source Devlin et al. (2010)

Table 2.5 Changes in health state for three conditions according to the PCHC, taking account of those with no problems

	Hernia	Veins	Cataract
Number with problems (% of those with problems)			
No change	53 (14.9%)	29 (13.0%)	99 (20.8%)
Improve	203 (57.0%)	148 (66.4%)	149 (31.4%)
Worsen	71 (19.9%)	34 (15.2%)	188 (39.6%)
Mixed change	29 (8.2%)	12 (5.4%)	39 (8.2%)
Total with problems	356 (82.8%)	223 (83.8%)	475 (66.8%)
No problems	74 (17.2%)	43 (16.2%)	236 (33.2%)

Source Devlin et al. (2010)

replacement operations a close second. Hernia and varicose vein repairs were much less successful, and cataract removals had a very low success rate, with more patients getting worse than improving—although the last of these should be interpreted carefully because the EQ-5D may not be capturing the kind of benefits that cataract operations provide. The numbers of patients who worsened or had no change show the same pattern.

One problem with this analysis is that 'No change' is confounded when patients record no problems according to any of the dimensions before treatment, because they are, according to the EQ-5D, healthy patients whose only alternative would be for their condition to worsen as a result of treatment. Recording no problems at all is rare for patients who have conditions serious enough to require a joint replacement but may occur for conditions whose need for treatment may not be fully captured by their EQ-5D profile. Table 2.5 shows for the three conditions to which this applies the PCHC taking into account those with no problems before surgery. In each case, this shows a slightly better performance than suggested by Table 2.4.

The advantage of the PCHC is that it provides a high-level summary of the nature of changes in health reported by patients, without the need to introduce any external scoring system or preference weighting.

The limitations of the PCHC are:

(i)   It focuses on whether there is improvement or worsening in self-reported health, and does not account for the magnitude of those changes. It does not differentiate between small improvements and big improvements (e.g., both a shift from level 5 to level 4, and a shift from level 5 to level 1, are counted as improvements).

(ii) It takes no account of whether the changes occur in dimensions that matter a lot to people or in dimensions that may be considered less important.

(iii) The PCHC will not be informative in cases where mixed changes dominate the changes in health self-reported by patients.

The PCHC can be extended to give information about the composition of differences between profiles according to how dimensions and levels differ. These are illustrated using newer data on hip replacement patients in the English NHS PROMs programme that was instituted following the pilot study referred to earlier, using simple graphs. They also show how data can be compared at different time periods. This could be adapted to compare, for example, patients in different populations.

First, Fig. 2.1 shows the PCHC for three years in graphical form.

Figure 2.2 shows which dimensions were improved for those patients whose PCHC category was 'Improved'

This shows that improvements were spread over all dimensions, but were most frequently found in Pain and Discomfort, followed by Usual Activities and Mobility,

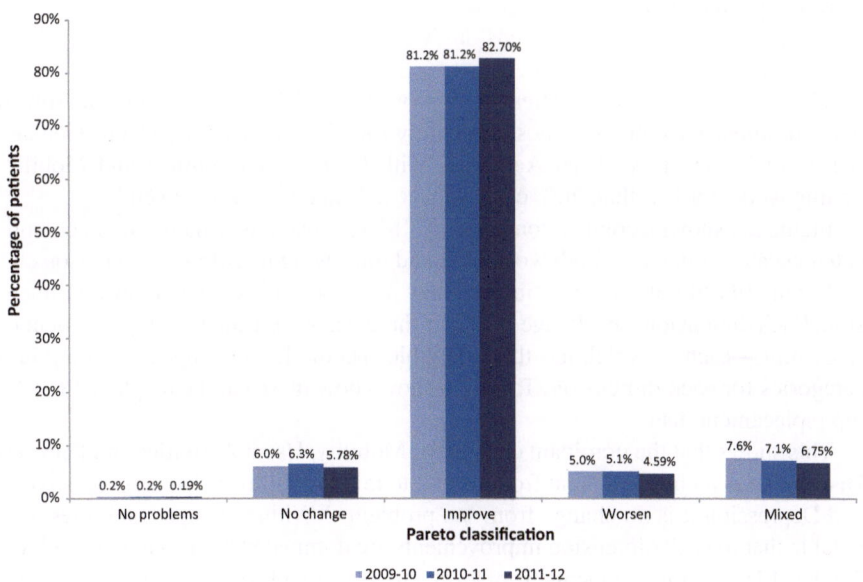

Fig. 2.1 The PCHC for hip replacement patients in the English NHS, 2009–12

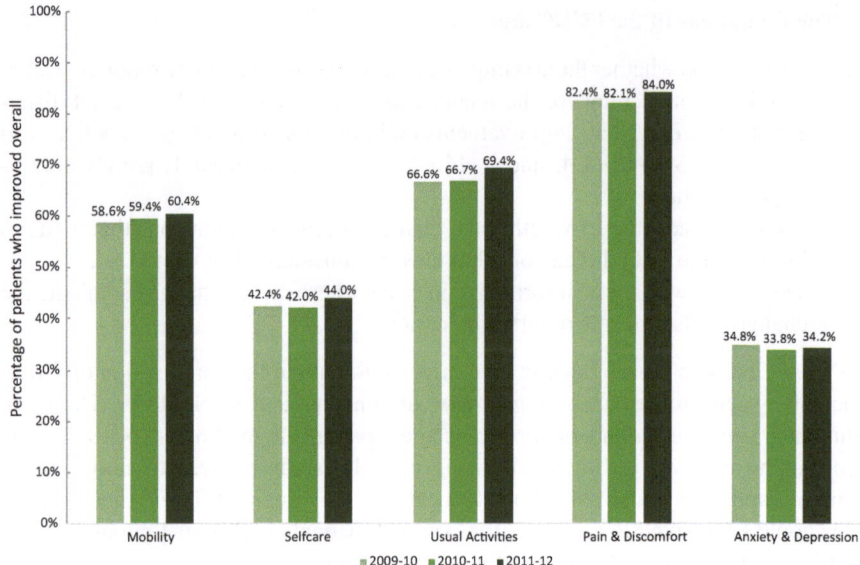

Fig. 2.2 Percentage of hip replacement patients who improved overall, by the dimensions in which they improved, English NHS 2009–2012

with Self-care and Anxiety and Depression improving for less than 50% of those who improved overall.

Figure 2.3 shows which dimensions were worsened for those patients whose PCHC category was 'Worsened'.

This shows the opposite pattern to improvements. Worsening health was spread over all dimensions, but was most frequently found in Anxiety and Depression and Self-Care followed by Usual Activities, with Pain and Discomfort and Mobility getting worse for less than 20% of those whose health was worse overall.

Figure 2.4 shows a comparison of PCHC 'Mixed' patients, which is more complicated because it involves both worsening and improving in different dimensions.

For the EQ-5D-3L, it is possible to show every possible change in every dimension. Each dimension can change in one of three ways—no change, improvement or worsening—each of which has three possible specific level changes, resulting in 9 categories for each dimension. Table 2.6 shows how these can be displayed for the hip replacement data.

This shows that the dominant change for Mobility, Usual Activities and Pain and Discomfort is an improvement from level 2 to level 1, but for Self-care and Anxiety and Depression it is no change from 'no problems.' Within change categories, it is notable that in each dimension improvements are dominated by a change from level 2 to level 1; that improvements from level 3 to level 1 and worsening from 1 to 3 are rare, reflecting the rarity of level 3 observations in the data set; and worsening from 2 to 3 is the most common amongst those who worsened overall in Usual Activities and Pain and Discomfort.

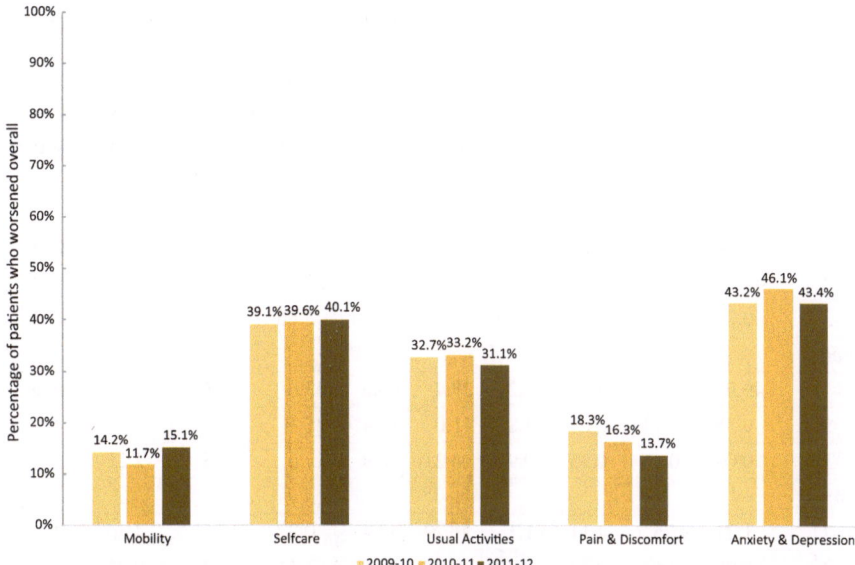

Fig. 2.3 Percentage of hip replacement patients whose health worsened overall, by the dimensions in which they worsened, English NHS 2009–12

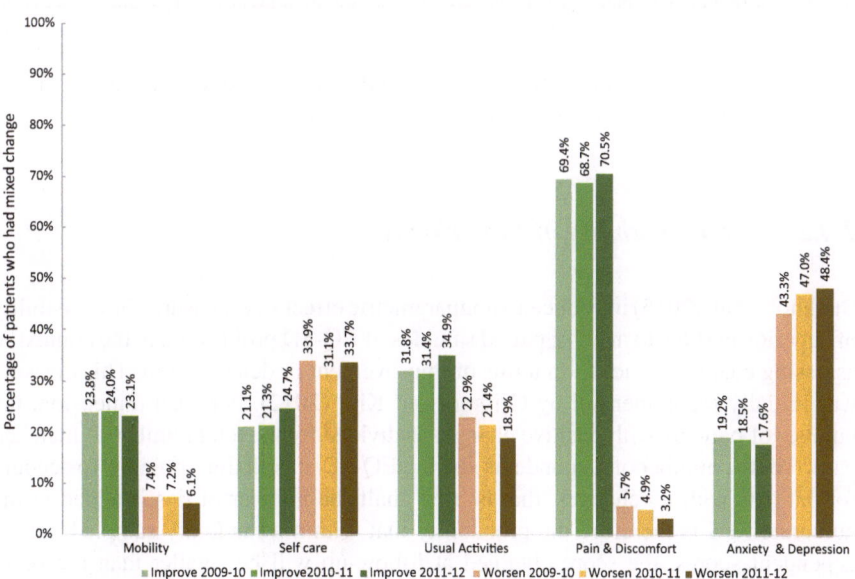

Fig. 2.4 Percentage of hip replacement patients who had a mixed change overall, by the dimensions in which they improved and worsened, English NHA 2009–12

Table 2.6 Changes in levels in each dimension for hip patients, NHS PROMs, 2009–10, percentages of total and of type of change

Change type	Mobility		Self-care		Usual activities		Pain and discomfort		Anxiety and depression	
	% total	% type	% total	% type	% total	% type	% total	% type	% total	% type
No change										
1–1	5.34	10.8	**40.2**	**67.6**	4.73	11.8	0.72	2.71	**52.8**	**81.5**
2–2	43.9	**89.1**	19.0	32.0	32.9	**82.0**	22.9	**86.5**	11.3	17.4
3–3	0.02	0.04	0.24	0.40	2.50	6.24	2.86	10.8	0.73	1.13
Better										
2–1	**49.0**	**99.1**	35.0	**97.2**	**39.4**	**69.6**	**33.6**	**46.5**	25.5	**85.6**
3–2	0.35	0.71	0.67	1.87	11.0	19.4	21.1	29.2	2.06	6.92
3–1	0.09	0.18	0.35	0.97	6.21	10.9	17.5	24.3	2.21	7.43
Worse										
1–2	1.21	**95.5**	4.11	**91.1**	1.29	38.4	0.22	16.5	4.26	**78.4**
2–3	0.06	4.52	0.33	7.25	1.97	**58.6**	1.11	**82.7**	0.93	17.1
1–3	0.00	0.00	0.08	1.68	0.10	3.06	0.01	0.85	0.25	4.55

% total = % of all in the relevant dimension; largest category highlighted in bold
% type = % of all in the change type in the relevant dimension; largest category highlighted in bold

Unfortunately, it is much more difficult to display the same analysis for the 5L version, as there are 25 possible categories for each dimension.

2.4.2   The Probability of Superiority

Buchholz et al. (2015) introduced a nonparametric effect size measure, the probability of superiority (PS), to analyse paired samples of EQ-5D profile data in the context of assessing changes in health in terms of improvement or deterioration. This measure was initially recommended by Grissom and Kim (2012). For each dimension, the number of patients with positive changes is divided by the total number of matched pairs (i.e. the number of respondents scoring EQ-5D at both time-points). To account for patients with no changes, that is 'ties', half the number of ties is added to the numerator. PS is therefore the probability that within a randomly sampled pair of dependent scores, the score obtained at follow-up will be smaller than the score obtained at baseline. It ranges from 0 to 1 and is

- <0.5 if more patients deteriorate than improve,
- = 0.5 if the same number of patients improve and deteriorate or do not change and
- >0.5 if more patients improve than deteriorate.

This is a further, useful way of examining the nature of change in EQ-5D data. A limitation is that it focuses on changes at the dimension level, rather than on how this combines at the patient level.

2.4.3   Health Profile Grid (HPG)

A further way of summarising changes in health in an EQ-5D data set is the Health Profile Grid (HPG), also introduced by Devlin et al. (2010). The HPG relies on profiles being ordered from best to worst. This can be done using a value set, a scoring system based on equally weighted dimensions and levels, or a scoring system based on the EQ VAS predicted from the profile (see Chap. 4).

The HPG plots the profiles between any two points in time. The example shown in Fig. 2.5, again taken from the English NHS PROMs pilot, shows profiles before and six months after hip replacement surgery. The rank ordering is determined by the EQ-5D-3L values according to the value set for the United Kingdom (Dolan et al. 1997). The PCHC category for each profile change is also shown.

The location of each point shows improvement and worsening according to the profiles' rank order. The 45° line represents 'no change'; the further above the line, the greater the improvement in health; below the line means health has worsened. The pattern of observations in the HPG in Fig. 2.5 suggests that most patients experience benefit from hip replacement surgery, as the observations lie predominantly

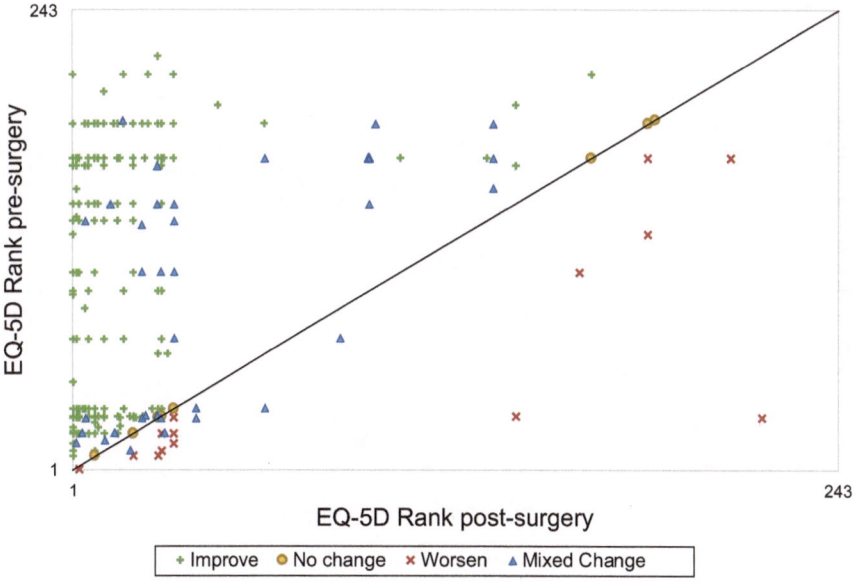

Fig. 2.5 Health profile grid for hip operations, English NHS

above the 45° line. There is a spread of health profiles from less to more severe before surgery, but a much narrower distribution after surgery, concentrated in the least severe profiles, with some outliers. The PCHC category adds to this by identifying cases where overall improvement and worsening of the patients' 'before' and 'after' profiles according to their rank are 'Mixed Change', that is they include both improvements in at least one dimension and worsening in at least one other. In these data, every mixed change case included only one dimension which changed in the opposite direction to the overall change according to the profiles' rank.

By contrast, the HPG shown in Fig. 2.6, for the English NHS PROMs pilot cataract surgery data, shows a much more mixed picture of improvements and worsening. The immediately obvious observation is that similar numbers improved and worsened. However, another feature is that most of those with the worst health profiles before surgery improved and most of those with the worst profiles after surgery had amongst the least severe health profiles before surgery. Unlike the clear-cut conclusions that may be drawn from the hip HPG, such a pattern suggests further investigation is required into the impact of cataract operations on patients' health-related quality of life (HRQoL).

Presenting the profiles in this manner can suggest clusters of patients, characterised by the nature of their profiles at time point 1, and the direction and magnitude of the change between the time-points. However, it is important not to rely on visual inspection alone to identify clusters, because some of the gaps that are apparent simply identify EQ-5D health profiles that are very infrequently observed, for example states having no problems in four dimensions and the worst state in the

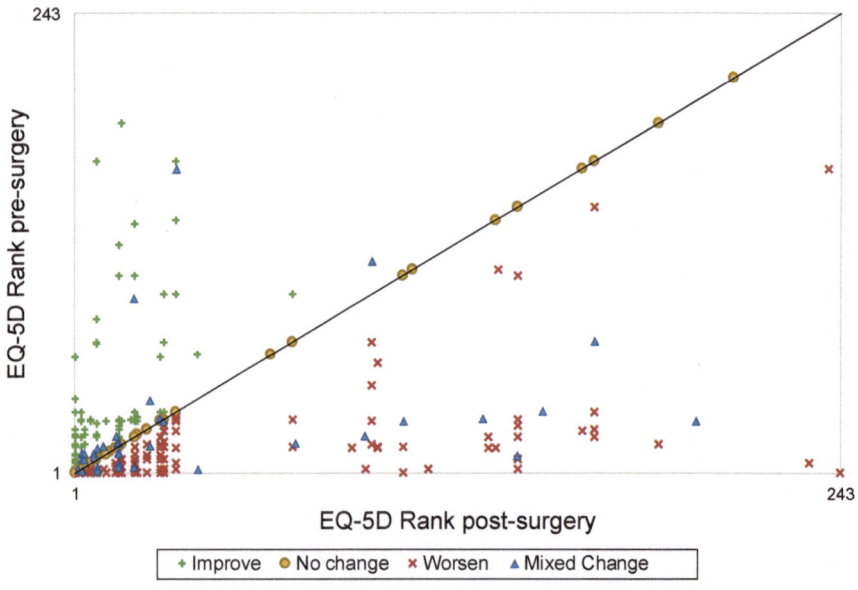

Fig. 2.6 Health profile grid for cataract operations, English NHS

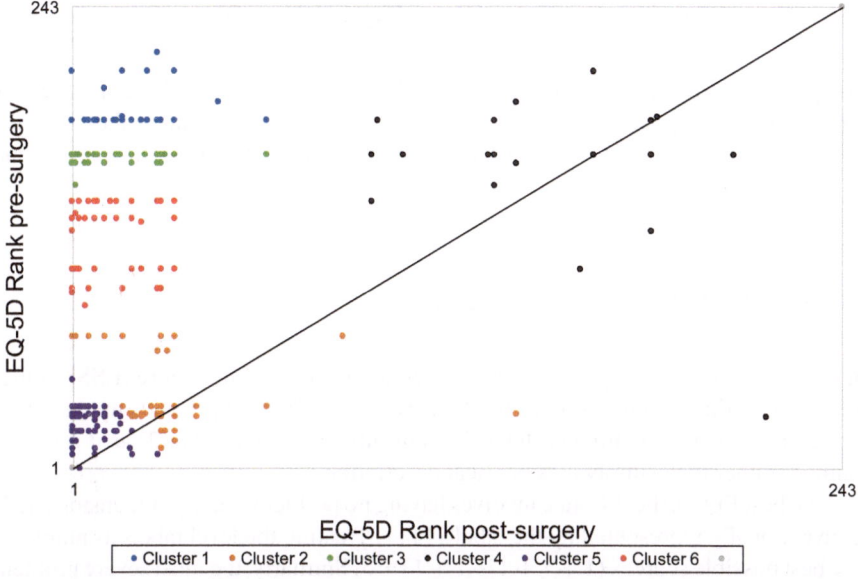

Fig. 2.7 Health profile grid showing clusters of changes in health for NHS hip replacement patients, using the k-means procedure

other. It is essential to test for these formally using statistical cluster analysis techniques. An example, with clusters identified using a k-means procedure, is shown in Fig. 2.7.

The numbers represent the 6 different clusters of patients identified. Most of the clusters seem to be identified as similar because of the patients similar pre-surgery profiles. Cluster 4 is of more interest, identifiable as the patients with worst health profiles after surgery. Also of interest is the comparison of clusters 2 and 5, with similar, relatively less severe profiles before surgery but with cluster 2 having more severe profiles after surgery. These observations could form the basis of further investigation into whether or not these are real clusters of clinical importance.

It is to possible to improve the appearance of the HPG and reduce the problem of artefactual gaps by including only those health states found within the data. It is also possible to take this further by including only the most frequently found profiles. In many data sets, only a few very common profiles are found, along with many rarer cases, so restricting the analysis to profiles covering, for example, 90% of all observations would be informative.

The advantage of the HPG is that it provides a ready means of displaying and examining the changes in health within a sample of patients. A limitation of the HPG is that it relies upon having a valid and appropriate means of ranking the EQ-5D profiles. The method used to rank the profiles may affect the HPG and the statistical identification of clusters.

2.5   Summarising the Severity of EQ-5D Profiles

It is sometimes useful to summarise the overall 'severity' of EQ-5D health states, by means other than generating weighted scores such as values. Because these involve information loss and hidden assumptions about the aggregation of dimensions and levels, they should be used with care.

2.5.1   The Level Sum Score (LSS)

It is possible to summarise a profile by calculating a Level Sum Score (LSS), sometimes misleadingly referred to as the 'misery score'. This simply adds up the levels on each dimension, treating each level's conventional label (1, 2 or 3) as if it were a number rather than simply a categorical description.

The best EQ-5D health state involves having no problems on any dimension and is conventionally represented by the label 11111. Treating the level labels as numbers, the best possible score is $(1 + 1 + 1 + 1 + 1) = 5$. Similarly, the most severe problem on any dimension has the label 3 for the EQ-5D-3L, so the LSS for the worst health state is $(3 + 3 + 3 + 3 + 3) = 15$. Every other health state on the EQ-5D-3L will have a level sum score between 5 (the best) and 15 (the worst 15), and as these are integer there are 11 possible scores; the larger the score, the worse the health state. For the EQ-5D-5L, the range is between 5 and 25 and there are 21 possible scores.

The LSS has been used as a crude measure of severity to gauge the validity of values obtained in valuation for studies for different health states. Figure 2.8 shows the relationship between the English value set for the EQ-5D-5L and the LSS (Devlin et al. 2018). This shows that, as the LSS increases (states get worse), the values decline.

However, the LSS has some important limitations as a means of summarising health states across dimensions and levels:

(i)   It's a very crude summary score—for example, the very different EQ-5D-3L profiles 22222, 33211 and 11233 all have the same level sum score (LSS = 10). The Dutch values for these profiles are 0.569, 0.350 and 0.009 respectively (Lamers et al. 2006).

(ii) Within the LSS scores, the weighted index values derived from profiles have very wide and overlapping ranges.

(iii) Each score contains a very different number of potential profiles: for example, in the EQ-5D-3L, LSS = 5 and LSS = 15 have just one profile each, but LSS = 10 contains 51 profiles. For the 5L, there are 381 profiles with LSS = 15, but just 5 profiles with a LSS = 6.

(iv) Giving equal weight to the dimensions and the difference between levels means the LSS is not free from value judgements—it makes a specific assumption about their relative importance (Parkin et al. 2010).

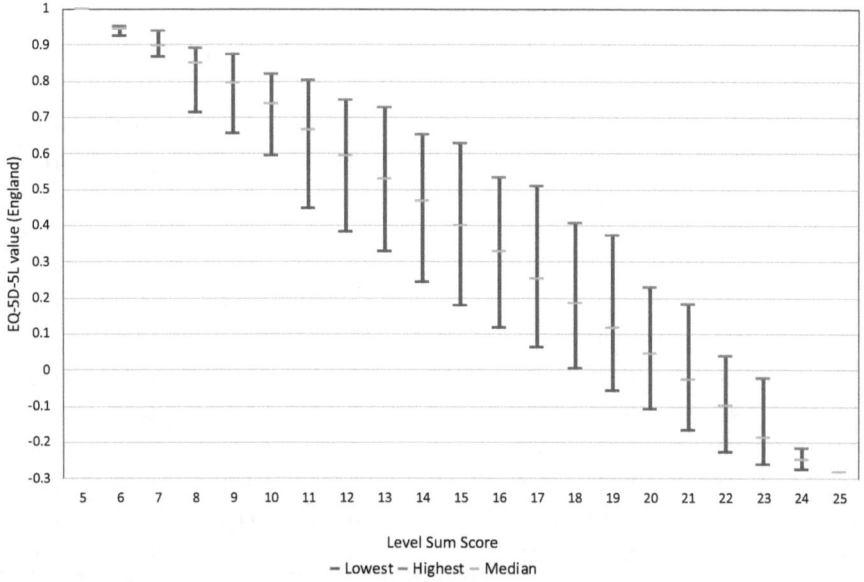

Fig. 2.8 EQ-5D-5L values (English value set) plotted against the LSS

These issues can be seen below, with respect to the EQ-5D-5L. Table 2.7 shows all possible LSSs for the EQ-5D-5L. It also shows descriptive statistics for the English value set for the EQ-5D-5L for all the different LSSs for the EQ-5D-5L. Although the mean and median values relate reasonably well to the order of the LSS, it does show big differences in the standard deviation. Importantly, it shows the overlap between the range of values for the different level summary scores. For example, the range for LSS = 15 includes the mean values of LSS = 12 and LSS = 18 and the lower or upper range respectively of LSS = 10 and LSS = 21. This issue can also be seen in Fig. 2.8. For these reasons, it is wrong to treat the LSS as ordinal.

2.5.2 The Level Frequency Score (LFS)

An alternative, although rarely used, means of summarising profile data is the level frequency score (LFS). The measure was proposed by Oppe and de Charro (2001) and used there to demonstrate the distribution of the EQ-5D-3L profiles in their data on the effects on HRQoL of a helicopter trauma team. The method characterises each health state by the frequency of levels at 1, 2 or 3 (for the EQ-5D-3L) or the frequency of levels at 1, 2, 3, 4 and 5 on the EQ-5D-5L. For example, in the EQ-5D-5L, the full health profile 11111 has 5, 1 s, no level 2, 3, 4 and 5 s, so the LFS is 50000; the worst health profile is 00005; profiles such as 31524 and 53412 would be 11111; 20 profiles such as 13211 have a LFS of 31100.

Table 2.7 Summary statistics for the EQ-5D-5L values (English value set) by all the different LSSs

Sum score	Number	Mean	Standard deviation	Median	Minimum	Maximum	Range
5	1	1.000	–	1.000	1.000	1.000	0.000
6	5	0.942	0.011	0.945	0.924	0.951	0.027
7	15	0.898	0.024	0.896	0.866	0.939	0.074
8	35	0.844	0.039	0.850	0.714	0.890	0.176
9	70	0.783	0.056	0.795	0.656	0.874	0.219
10	121	0.722	0.063	0.737	0.594	0.819	0.225
11	185	0.660	0.068	0.667	0.447	0.802	0.355
12	255	0.595	0.074	0.593	0.384	0.747	0.363
13	320	0.530	0.079	0.530	0.329	0.728	0.400
14	365	0.463	0.081	0.467	0.241	0.652	0.410
15	381	0.396	0.083	0.399	0.179	0.628	0.449
16	365	0.327	0.085	0.329	0.118	0.533	0.415
17	320	0.258	0.085	0.254	0.062	0.509	0.446
18	255	0.189	0.083	0.186	0.003	0.407	0.403
19	185	0.118	0.083	0.118	−0.057	0.372	0.430
20	121	0.045	0.079	0.045	−0.107	0.228	0.335
21	70	−0.025	0.073	−0.026	−0.165	0.181	0.346
22	35	−0.098	0.068	−0.099	−0.226	0.037	0.263
23	15	−0.173	0.066	−0.185	−0.261	−0.024	0.237
24	5	−0.245	0.026	−0.246	−0.276	−0.218	0.058
25	1	−0.281	–	−0.281	−0.281	−0.281	0.000

Oppe and de Charro used the LFS to show the way in which the EQ-5D-3L values data observed in their data (using the UK EQ-5D-3L value set) were distributed over the various EQ-5D-3L profiles (see Table 2.8).

The distribution of EQ-5D-5L profiles by LFS is provided in an Appendix to this chapter.

2.6   Analysing the Informativity of EQ-5D Profile Data

2.6.1   Shannon Indices

Shannon's indices, originally developed to analyse the information content of strings of text, are widely used in the ecology literature to measure how many species are observed and how evenly animals, or plants are spread over the various categories. It has also been applied widely in assessing distributional characteristics of the EQ-5D

Table 2.8 Number of observations in the LFS according to the UK EQ-5D-3L values

Value	0 1 4	0 2 3	0 4 1	0 5 0	1 2 2	1 3 1	1 4 0	2 1 2	2 2 1	2 3 0	3 1 1	3 2 0	4 1 0	5 0 0	Total
−0.484	1														1
−0.166		1													1
−0.016			1												1
−0.003					3										3
0.030					2										2
0.055						1									1
0.082			2												2
0.088						3									3
0.101								2							2
0.150					1										1
0.189			1												1
0.255									1						1
0.291											1				1
0.293						2									2
0.329									1						1
0.516				6											6
0.585							2								2
0.587							9								9
0.620							15								16
0.656										2					2
0.689										13					13
0.691										25					25
0.710										1					1
0.725												5			5
0.727												15			15
0.743										2					2
0.744												1			1
0.760												9			9
0.796													13		13
0.812												5			5
0.814												3			3
0.848													3		3
0.850													2		2
0.883													4		4
1.000														33	33
Total	1	1	4	6	6	6	27	2	2	43	1	38	22	33	192

Source Taken from a EuroQol scientific plenary paper which preceded the subsequent journal articles

(Buchholz et al. 2018), where the categories of interest are EQ-5D profiles and we are interested in a summary measure of how evenly respondents to EQ-5D questionnaires are spread over the profiles defined by the descriptive system. The main application of the Shannon indices has been to compare informational richness and evenness of dimensions, either comparing the EQ-5D-3L with the EQ-5D-5L or to compare similar dimensions between different generic health status instruments (Janssen et al. 2007). It is also possible to apply the Shannon indices to distributions of health profiles.

The Shannon index is defined as:

$$H' = -\sum_{i=1}^{C} p_i \log_2 p_i$$

where H' represents the absolute amount of informativity captured, C is the total number of possible categories (levels or profiles), and $p_i = n_i/N$, the proportion of observations in the ith category ($i = 1,..., C$), where n_i is the observed number of scores (responses) in category i and N is the total sample size. The higher the index H' is, the more information is captured by the dimension or instrument. In the case of a uniform (rectangular) distribution (i.e., $p_i = p^*$ for all i), the optimal amount of information is captured and H' has reached its maximum (H'max) which equals $\log_2 C$. If the number of categories (C) is increased, H'max increases accordingly, but H' will only increase if the newly added categories are actually used. The Shannon Evenness index (J') exclusively reflects the evenness (rectangularity) of a distribution, regardless of the number of categories, and is defined as: $J' = H'/H'$max. Variance of the Shannon index can be calculated as described by Janssen et al. (2007) and accordingly standard errors and 95% confidence intervals can be calculated.

The Shannon indices are purely descriptive measures of the informational richness and evenness of a classification system and have no relation to the content, meaning, or clinical relevance of what the instrument aims to measure. Both the Shannon index and the Shannon Evenness index are needed to make a useful interpretation of the measurement scale.

2.6.2   Health State Density Curve (HSDC)

Zamora et al. (2018) introduced a graphical means of depicting the nature of the distribution of EQ-5D profiles, the health state density curve (HSDC). This draws on an analogy with the Lorenz curve in describing an income distribution. The cumulative frequency of health states is compared against the cumulative frequency of the sample or population. A 45° line means that the observed health states are completely evenly spread across the sample: 10% of the sample accounts for 10% of the health states; 50% of the sample accounts for 50% of the health states, and so on.

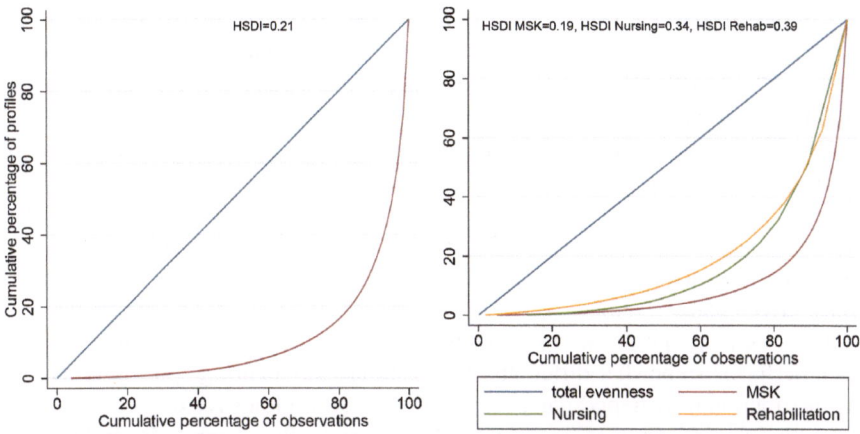

Fig. 2.9 HSDC for EQ-5D-5L profiles from Cambridgeshire NHS patients

A concentrated distribution—that is, where relatively few profiles are reported and are common to a large proportion of the sample—will be show as a curve which lies below the 45° line. The more unevenly distributed the profile data, the further below the diagonal line the HSDC will be. In the extreme, where just one profile is reported by all members of the sample, the HSDC will take a right-angled shape.

Figure 2.9 shows the HSDC for patients from three groups of patients, and overall, from Cambridgeshire NHS in the UK. This shows that for all patients, observed profiles are not evenly distributed, that is a small number of profiles accounts for a relatively large share of the observations. The musculoskeletal patients had the most concentrated data.

The HSDC provides a simple means of illustrating this property of a profile data set, in a manner that facilitates comparisons between data sets. It has limitations. As with Lorenz curves, where two curves cross (as is the case with rehabilitation and nursing data shown in Fig. 2.9), there is no unequivocal way of declaring one data set to be more concentrated than another. It also does not tell us which profiles are the most commonly self-reported. Therefore, the HSDC is best seen as a complement to the information from the cumulative frequency of profiles.

2.6.3 Health State Density Index (HSDI) and Other Related Indices

In the analysis of income distribution, the Lorenz curve is often accompanied by the Gini coefficient, which describes the extent of inequality which is apparent as the area between the diagonal line and the curve, divided by the entire area underneath the diagonal. In a similar way, an index can be calculated to summarise the inequality of observed health state profiles. Zamora et al. (2018) introduce a broadly similar summary measure, the Health State Density Index (HSDI). HSDI has a value of 1 where there is total equality, that is where there are the same number of patients in each profile, and HSDI = 0 for total inequality, that is where one profile accounts for all the observations.

The HSDI allows the degree of concentration in self-reported health to be compared both between different sets of patients and between different instruments, for example the 3 and 5 level versions of the EQ-5D. Zamora et al. (2018) use the HSDC to compare the EQ-5D-3L and EQ-5D-5L, their respective HSDIs indicating the advantages of the 5L in differentiating between patients and yielding less concentrated data.

The specific properties of the HSDI may be compared with the Shannon' indices. Each performs somewhat differently as a measure in capturing specific aspects of the distribution of patients' data, such as the concentration over the most common states, and the influence of 'rare' states. For example, the Shannon index (absolute and relative) is not sensitive to random variations but decreases slowly with "rare health states". The HSDI decreases slowly with random variations and is strongly affected by infrequently observed health states with large decreases towards zero (total inequality). For more detail see Zamora et al. (2018).

Appendix: Analysis of the LFS for the EQ-5D-5L

For the EQ-5D-5L, the LFS has a total of 102 possible scores, from 00005 (for the worst profile 55555) through to 50000 (no problem on any dimension, state 11111). Like the LSS, a problem with the LFS is that LFSs contain an uneven number of profiles. For example, LFS = 50000 and LFS = 00005 each contain 1 profile, whereas LFS = 11111 (meaning: any health profile containing one level 1, one level 2, one level 3, one level 4 and one level 5) represents 120 different EQ-5D-5L profiles. Table 2.9 is a full list of the possible values for the LFS.

Table 2.9 Distribution of the EQ-5D-5L profiles by LFS

LFS	Freq.	%	Cum. (%)	LFS	Freq.	%	Cum. (%)	LFS	Freq.	%	Cum (%)
11111	120	3.84	3.84	20120	30	0.96	63.36	00230	10	0.32	91.52
01112	60	1.92	5.76	20201	30	0.96	64.32	00302	10	0.32	91.84
01121	60	1.92	7.68	20210	30	0.96	65.28	00320	10	0.32	92.16
01211	60	1.92	9.6	21002	30	0.96	66.24	02003	10	0.32	92.48
02111	60	1.92	11.52	21020	30	0.96	67.2	02030	10	0.32	92.8
10112	60	1.92	13.44	21200	30	0.96	68.16	02300	10	0.32	93.12
10121	60	1.92	15.36	22001	30	0.96	69.12	03002	10	0.32	93.44
10211	60	1.92	17.28	22010	30	0.96	70.08	03020	10	0.32	93.76
11012	60	1.92	19.2	22100	30	0.96	71.04	03200	10	0.32	94.08
11021	60	1.92	21.12	00113	20	0.64	71.68	20003	10	0.32	94.4
11102	60	1.92	23.04	00131	20	0.64	72.32	20030	10	0.32	94.72
11120	60	1.92	24.96	00311	20	0.64	72.96	20300	10	0.32	95.04
11201	60	1.92	26.88	01013	20	0.64	73.6	23000	10	0.32	95.36
11210	60	1.92	28.8	01031	20	0.64	74.24	30002	10	0.32	95.68
12011	60	1.92	30.72	01103	20	0.64	74.88	30020	10	0.32	96
12101	60	1.92	32.64	01130	20	0.64	75.52	30200	10	0.32	96.32
12110	60	1.92	34.56	01301	20	0.64	76.16	32000	10	0.32	96.64
20111	60	1.92	36.48	01310	20	0.64	76.8	00014	5	0.16	96.8
21011	60	1.92	38.4	03011	20	0.64	77.44	00041	5	0.16	96.96
21101	60	1.92	40.32	03101	20	0.64	78.08	00104	5	0.16	97.12
21110	60	1.92	42.24	03110	20	0.64	78.72	00140	5	0.16	97.28
00122	30	0.96	43.2	10013	20	0.64	79.36	00401	5	0.16	97.44
00212	30	0.96	44.16	10031	20	0.64	80	00410	5	0.16	97.6
00221	30	0.96	45.12	10103	20	0.64	80.64	01004	5	0.16	97.76
01022	30	0.96	46.08	10130	20	0.64	81.28	01040	5	0.16	97.92
01202	30	0.96	47.04	10301	20	0.64	81.92	01400	5	0.16	98.08
01220	30	0.96	48	10310	20	0.64	82.56	04001	5	0.16	98.24
02012	30	0.96	48.96	11003	20	0.64	83.2	04010	5	0.16	98.4
02021	30	0.96	49.92	11030	20	0.64	83.84	04100	5	0.16	98.56
02102	30	0.96	50.88	11300	20	0.64	84.48	10004	5	0.16	98.72
02120	30	0.96	51.84	13001	20	0.64	85.12	10040	5	0.16	98.88
02201	30	0.96	52.8	13010	20	0.64	85.76	10400	5	0.16	99.04

Table 2.9 (continued)

LFS	Freq.	%	Cum. (%)	LFS	Freq.	%	Cum. (%)	LFS	Freq.	%	Cum (%)
02210	30	0.96	53.76	13100	20	0.64	86.4	14000	5	0.16	99.2
10022	30	0.96	54.72	30011	20	0.64	87.04	40001	5	0.16	99.36
10202	30	0.96	55.68	30101	20	0.64	87.68	40010	5	0.16	99.52
10220	30	0.96	56.64	30110	20	0.64	88.32	40100	5	0.16	99.68
12002	30	0.96	57.6	31001	20	0.64	88.96	41000	5	0.16	99.84
12020	30	0.96	58.56	31010	20	0.64	89.6	00005	1	0.03	99.87
12200	30	0.96	59.52	31100	20	0.64	90.24	00050	1	0.03	99.9
20012	30	0.96	60.48	00023	10	0.32	90.56	00500	1	0.03	99.94
20021	30	0.96	61.44	00032	10	0.32	90.88	05000	1	0.03	99.97
20102	30	0.96	62.4	00203	10	0.32	91.2	50000	1	0.03	100

Table 2.10 shows how the LFS could be used to analyse the characteristics of an EQ-5D-5L value set, using data from the English value set (Devlin et al. 2018). It shows the mean and median values for each LFS.

Table 2.10 Summary statistics of EQ-5D-5L values by LFS

LFS	Mean	Median	LFS	Mean	Median	LFS	Mean	Median
00005	−0.285	−0.285	02120	0.362	0.359	12101	0.543	0.535
00014	−0.247	−0.246	02201	0.461	0.452	12110	0.581	0.588
00023	−0.209	−0.209	02210	0.499	0.508	12200	0.718	0.717
00032	−0.171	−0.170	02300	0.637	0.637	13001	0.564	0.551
00041	−0.133	−0.134	03002	0.307	0.314	13010	0.602	0.609
00050	−0.095	−0.095	03011	0.345	0.348	13100	0.740	0.737
00104	−0.109	−0.099	03020	0.383	0.378	14000	0.762	0.760
00113	−0.071	−0.071	03101	0.483	0.473	20003	0.229	0.221
00122	−0.033	−0.031	03110	0.521	0.529	20012	0.267	0.262
00131	0.005	0.008	03200	0.659	0.659	20021	0.305	0.300
00140	0.043	0.037	04001	0.505	0.490	20030	0.343	0.349
00203	0.067	0.062	04010	0.543	0.553	20102	0.405	0.413
00212	0.105	0.093	04100	0.680	0.680	20111	0.443	0.448
00221	0.143	0.140	05000	0.702	0.702	20120	0.481	0.476
00230	0.181	0.184	10004	−0.028	−0.011	20201	0.581	0.570
00302	0.243	0.247	10013	0.010	0.019	20210	0.619	0.628

(continued)

Table 2.10 (continued)

LFS	Mean	Median	LFS	Mean	Median	LFS	Mean	Median
00311	0.281	0.285	10022	0.048	0.051	20300	0.756	0.756
00320	0.319	0.316	10031	0.086	0.082	21002	0.426	0.439
00401	0.418	0.408	10040	0.124	0.113	21011	0.464	0.466
00410	0.456	0.462	10103	0.148	0.138	21020	0.503	0.498
00500	0.594	0.594	10112	0.186	0.181	21101	0.602	0.591
01004	−0.087	−0.073	10121	0.224	0.222	21110	0.640	0.651
01013	−0.049	−0.049	10130	0.262	0.264	21200	0.778	0.777
01022	−0.011	−0.007	10202	0.324	0.331	22001	0.624	0.612
01031	0.027	0.024	10211	0.362	0.366	22010	0.662	0.673
01040	0.065	0.054	10220	0.400	0.393	22100	0.800	0.797
01103	0.088	0.083	10301	0.499	0.490	23000	0.821	0.819
01112	0.126	0.116	10310	0.537	0.544	30002	0.486	0.495
01121	0.164	0.157	10400	0.675	0.674	30011	0.524	0.526
01130	0.202	0.206	11003	0.170	0.164	30020	0.562	0.556
01202	0.264	0.269	11012	0.208	0.203	30101	0.662	0.647
01211	0.302	0.307	11021	0.246	0.243	30110	0.700	0.711
01220	0.340	0.335	11030	0.284	0.289	30200	0.838	0.838
01301	0.440	0.428	11102	0.345	0.357	31001	0.683	0.670
01310	0.478	0.486	11111	0.383	0.388	31010	0.721	0.737
01400	0.616	0.616	11120	0.421	0.415	31100	0.859	0.861
02003	0.110	0.103	11201	0.521	0.510	32000	0.881	0.883
02012	0.148	0.144	11210	0.559	0.566	40001	0.743	0.726
02021	0.186	0.177	11300	0.697	0.696	40010	0.781	0.793
02030	0.224	0.229	12002	0.367	0.378	40100	0.919	0.920
02102	0.286	0.293	12011	0.405	0.407	41000	0.940	0.942
02111	0.324	0.328	12020	0.443	0.436	50000	1.000	1.000

The following chart (Fig. 2.10) shows how the EVS and LFS are related. As with the LSS, this gives an indication of the general validity of a value set, in that there are no patterns that indicate that a value set takes perverse or other undesirable characteristics.

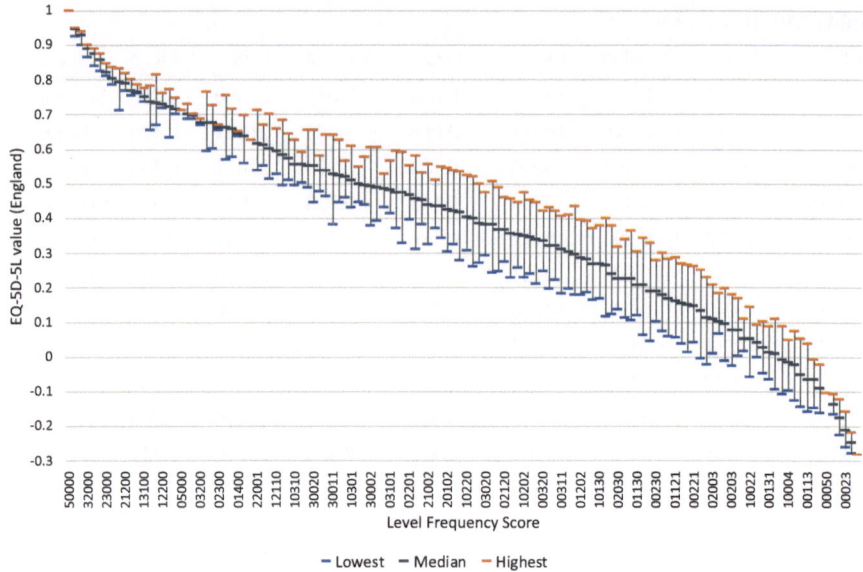

Fig. 2.10 EQ-5D-5L values (English value set) plotted against the LFS

References

Buchholz I, Janssen MF, Kohlmann T, Feng YS (2018) A systematic review of studies comparing the measurement properties of the three-level and five-level versions of the EQ-5D. Pharmacoecon 36(6):645–661

Buchholz I, Thielker K, Feng YS, Kupatz P, Kohlmann T (2015) Measuring changes in health over time using the EQ-5D 3L and 5L: a head-to-head comparison of measurement properties and sensitivity to change in a German inpatient rehabilitation sample. Qual Life Res 24(4):829–835

Devlin N, Parkin D, Browne J (2010) Using the EQ-5D as a performance measurement tool in the NHS. Health Econ 19(8):886–905

Devlin N, Shah K, Feng Y, Mulhern B, van Hout B (2018) Valuing health-related quality of life: an EQ-5D-5L value set for England. Health Econ 27(1):7–22

Dolan P (1997) Modeling valuations for EuroQol health states. Med Care 35(11):1095–1108

Feng Y, Devlin N, Herdman M (2015) Assessing the health of the general population in England: how do the three- and five-level versions of EQ-5D compare? Health Qual Life Outcomes 13:171

Grissom RJ, Kim JJ (2012) Effect sizes for research: univariate and multivariate applications, 2nd edn. Taylor & Francis, New York

Herdman M, Gudex C, Lloyd A, Janssen MF, Kind P, Parkin D, Bonsel GJ, Badia X (2011) Development and preliminary testing of the new five-level version of EQ-5D (EQ-5D-5L). Qual Life Res 20(10):1727–1736

Janssen MF, Birnie E, Bonsel GJ (2007) Evaluating the discriminatory power of EQ-5D, HUI2 and HUI3 in a US general population survey using Shannon's indices. Qual Life Res 16(5):895–904

Janssen MF, Bonsel GJ, Luo N (2018) Is EQ-5D-5L better than EQ-5D-3L? A head-to-head comparison of descriptive systems and value sets from seven countries. Pharmacoecon 36(6):675–697

Lamers LM, McDonnell J, Stalmeier PFM, Krabbe PFM, Busschbach JJV (2006) The Dutch tariff: results and arguments for an effective design for national EQ-5D valuation studies. Health Econ 15(10):1121–1132

Oppe M, Devlin N, Black N (2011) Comparison of the underlying constructs of the EQ-5D and Oxford Hip Score: implications for mapping. Value Health 14(6):884–891

Oppe S, De Charro FT (2001) The effect of medical care by a helicopter trauma team on the probability of survival and the quality of life of hospitalised victims. Accid Anal Prev 33(1):129–138

Parkin D, Devlin N, Feng Y (2016) What determines the shape of an EQ-5D index distribution? Med Decis Making 36(8):941–951

Parkin D, Rice N, Devlin N (2010) Statistical analysis of EQ-5D profiles: does the use of value sets bias inference? Med Decis Making 30(5):556–565

Zamora B, Parkin D, Feng Y, Bateman A, Herdman M, Devlin N (2018) New methods for analysing the distribution of EQ-5D observations. OHE Research Paper. www.ohe.org/publications/new-methods-analysing-distribution-eq-5d-observations

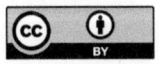

Chapter 3
Analysis of EQ VAS Data

The aims of this chapter are

- to explain what is measured by the EQ VAS, and how that affects analysis of EQ VAS data; and
- to demonstrate ways in which EQ VAS data can be analysed and reported.

3.1 Interpreting the EQ VAS

It is important when analysing EQ VAS data to understand the nature of this element of the EQ-5D questionnaire and the measurement properties that it has. (For a more detailed discussion, see Feng et al. 2014.) The EQ VAS has a unique design that does not conform to conventional Visual Analogue Scale (VAS) formats, and the widely-observed properties that VAS data have therefore do not automatically apply to EQ VAS data. It has some features that conventionally belong to a 'rating scale' but again, because it has an unconventional design, the properties that rating scale data have may also not apply.

A conventional VAS is a straight line of a specified length with verbal descriptors at each end stating the meaning attached to the end points, without any demarcations of the line or numeric labels at any point. The EQ VAS is also a line that has end-point descriptors, but it also demarcates the line in units of ones and tens, and places number labels on the tens markers. This format for the line is closer to a 'numerical rating scale', but such scales usually attach a number to every marker, have many fewer markers, and often do not have verbal end-point descriptors.

The versions of the EQ VAS contained in the EQ-5D-3L and EQ-5D-5L are also unconventional in how the scores are recorded by respondents. For the EQ-5D-3L version, the method of drawing a line from a box that states 'Your own health state today' to the scale (see Fig. 1.4, Chap. 1) is unique; it is a feature that was included

N. Devlin et al., *Methods for Analysing and Reporting EQ-5D Data*,
https://doi.org/10.1007/978-3-030-47622-9_3

for reasons related to the historical development of the EQ-5D[1] rather than evidence about the best way for respondents to record EQ VAS scores (Feng et al. 2014). The EQ-5D-5L uses a more conventional means of recording the score on the line (by marking a cross) but asks respondents also to record the score separately as a number. The aim of this is to overcome problems of imprecise marking on the line, but this introduces the possibility that respondents may respond primarily to the direct numeric estimate and are therefore undertaking a different measurement task, 'magnitude estimation', data from which may also have different properties to VAS and rating scale data.

The measurement properties that result from this, and therefore the kinds of statistical analysis that are permitted, are therefore not entirely clear. It is reasonable to assume that the resulting scores are at least ordinal. The line's design strongly suggests that the respondent is invited to supply interval level data, which is also the intention of magnitude estimation. The provision of a true zero and maximum even suggests providing scores that have ratio level properties. However, those who complete the VAS may in practice not respond to the visual stimuli provided in exactly this way. The evidence is mixed, with some studies finding reasonable interval scale properties; however, EQ VAS responses have very often been found to exhibit 'end aversion', which suggests that the data cannot be truly interval, though it is possible that a transformation could be estimated to repair this.

Another consideration is that, as with all health-related quality of life (HRQoL) measurement methods, EQ-VAS responses may not be interpersonally comparable. For example, the end-point labels may mean different things to different respondents, and the meaning that they attach to different numbers may also differ (Devlin et al. 2019).

The guidelines for analysis of EQ VAS data below assume that the numerical values given to the EQ VAS behave as if they have at least an interval scale and are interpersonally comparable, such that it is meaningful to calculate descriptive statistics for a sample or population, such as means; to apply hypothesis testing, such as t-tests of differences in means; and to use estimation procedures, such as regression analysis. However, if there is evidence to suggest that the EQ VAS data are ordinal, then non-parametric versions of the descriptive and inferential statistics described below should be used.

It is also the case that EQ VAS data often exhibit digit preference, which is a tendency to choose numbers ending with 0 and to a lesser extent 5, rather than any others. In the context of sample or population data, this phenomenon may be treated as a lack of precision rather than the existence of bias.

Before beginning to analyse EQ VAS data that have been collected via paper questionnaires for the EQ-5D-3L, it is important to check how those data have been coded. Recall, from Chap. 1, that there are particular issues relating to the range of approaches which respondents have been observed to use in completing the EQ VAS

---

[1]Specifically, the EQ VAS was initially included as a warm-up task in studies to obtain VAS valuations for EQ-5D health states, and the format of the EQ VAS reflects the VAS which was used in those valuation tasks.

in the EQ-5D-3L questionnaire. These may not strictly comply with the instructions but nevertheless represent valid responses. The EQ VAS in the EQ-5D-3L will, in future, be made consistent with the EQ VAS in the EQ-5D-5L, so this issue will no longer arise, but does apply to historic data sets.

3.2 Simple Descriptive Statistics and Inference

With respect to summary measures, the distribution of EQ VAS data within a sample can be reported using a full range of descriptive statistics, such as minimums, maximums, means, medians, quartiles, standard deviations, interquartile ranges, skewness and kurtosis. Descriptions of relationships between EQ VAS data and other variables can also be reported, such as correlation coefficients. These may be subject to appropriate hypothesis testing using, for example, a t-test to test for differences between means or for the significance of a correlation coefficient. Similarly, EQ VAS data can be used for estimation, either as a dependent or independent variable.

The following example uses publicly available data from the Patient Reported Outcome Measures (PROMs) programme of the English National Health Service (NHS) (Devlin et al. 2010). It shows data collected from 38,187 patients before and after they had hip replacement surgery in 2010–11. The following Table 3.1 shows a range of descriptive statistics.

Because the raw data are recorded as integers, it is important to ensure that the figures reported do not have spurious accuracy. In this table, the median and the mode (in this case, there is only one) retain their integer format. The median might be presented to one decimal place, reflecting the possible values that it could take, but because of digit preference a value ending in 0.5 will be rarely observed. Other statistics are presented to three significant figures, since it is unlikely that greater

Table 3.1 EQ VAS score for 38,187 patients before and after they had hip replacement surgery in the English NHS, 2010–11

EQ VAS score	Before surgery	After surgery
Mean	65.3	74.4
Standard error	0.116	0.102
Median	70	80
Mode	80	90
Standard deviation	21.7	19.34
Kurtosis	−0.110	1.37
Skewness	−0.672	−1.17
Minimum	0	0
Maximum	100	100
Range	100	100
Observations	34,716	35,762
Missing (percent)	3,471 (9.09%)	2,425 (6.35%)

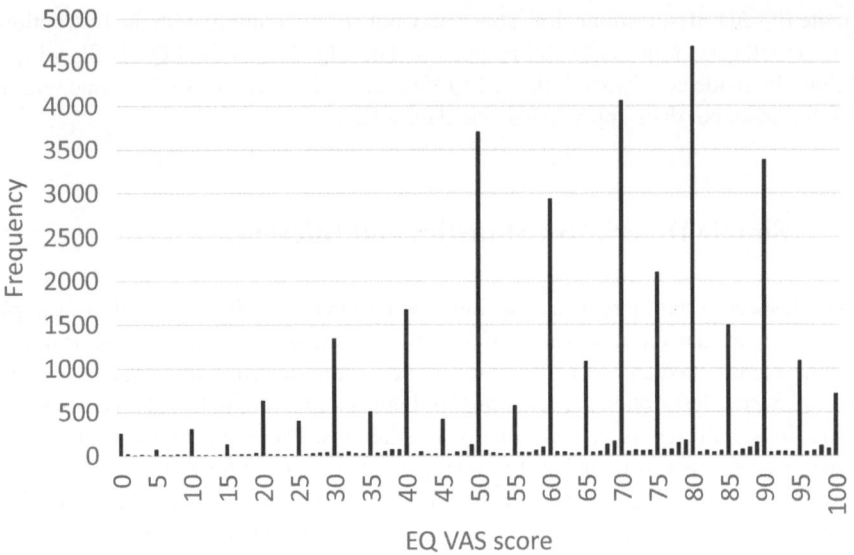

Fig. 3.1 EQ VAS scores for hip replacement patients before surgery, English NHS 2010–11

precision than this is either necessary or justified. It is also good practice to report the number and percentage of missing values.

It is also informative to report the full distribution of individual EQ VAS data points, especially graphically. A table showing the frequency of observations taking values from the full range of possible scores is possible but may not be very informative about key features of the distribution and will be affected by the issue of digit preference. It is most useful to use a graphical display, particularly spike plots. An example is shown in Fig. 3.1, again using the before-surgery hip replacement data.

This plot not only shows the shape and central tendency of the distribution, but also the extent of digit preference.

It is possible to reduce frequency tables to categories containing ranges, which makes them more easily read. However, end points for ranges should be chosen carefully, as this may affect the visual appearance of the distribution. It is misleading, for example, to define ranges such as 0–4, 5–9, 10–14 etc., as observations such as 9 are more like 10 than 5, for example. It is better to define ranges such that they cover a midpoint, specifically multiples of 5 and 10. However, at the ends of the distribution it may be better to display individual scores for those below the range around 5 (0, 1 and 2) and above the range around 95 (98, 99 and 100) rather than assume they are all representative of 0 and 100. The following Table 3.2 and Fig. 3.2 show this procedure for the before-surgery hip replacement data.

Table 3.3 shows analyses of the similarity and differences between the two observations. In this example, the two EQ VAS scores (before and after surgery) are paired, but it would be possible to undertake similar analyses for unpaired data.

Table 3.2 EQ VAS scores for hip replacement patients before surgery, English NHS 2010–11

Range	Mid-point	Frequency	Range	Mid-point	Frequency
0	0	253	58–62	60	3161
1	1	15	63–67	65	1202
2	2	3	68–72	70	4438
3–7	5	87	73–77	75	2324
8–12	10	335	78–82	80	5060
13–17	15	151	83–87	85	1677
18–22	20	683	88–92	90	3694
23–27	25	444	93–97	95	1262
28–32	30	1458	98	98	113
33–37	35	611	99	99	77
38–42	40	1855	100	100	707
43–47	45	491	Total observed		34,716
48–52	50	3947	Missing		3,471
53–57	55	668	Total sample		38,187

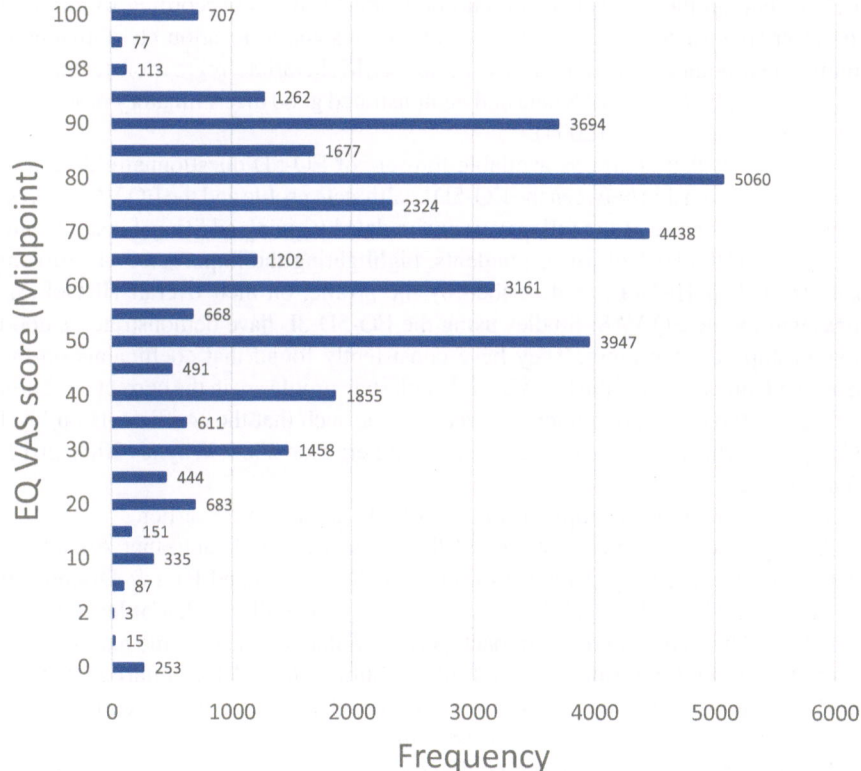

Fig. 3.2 Mid-point EQ VAS scores for hip replacement patients before surgery, English NHS 2010–11

Table 3.3 EQ VAS scores for hip replacement patients before and after surgery, English NHS 2010–11

	EQ VAS score	
	Before surgery	After surgery
Mean	65.4	74.6
Standard Deviation	21.7	19.2
Observations	32 712	
Missing values	5 475 (14.3%)	
Difference in means		
t-statistic	−69.94	
p value (one- and two-tail)	<0.001	
Pearson Correlation	0.33	

3.3 Modelling Determinants of EQ VAS Scores

It will usually be of interest in analysing EQ VAS data to examine the impact of other variables on the EQ VAS scores. In the example above, a before-and-after comparison was made between scores obtained from the same people at two time periods, but similar comparisons could be made for people according to different characteristics such as age, gender, social circumstances, location etc. Obviously, multivariate comparisons could also be made. Multivariate regression techniques have been applied to EQ VAS data and demonstrated good discriminatory properties, for example Parkin et al. (2004).

An analysis that is always available to users of EQ-5D questionnaire data is to model the relationship between the EQ-5D health state profile and the EQ VAS scores. This makes good use of the full questionnaire data by giving additional insights into the nature of the HRQoL of respondents, highlighting the importance of different aspects of their HRQoL, as described by the profile, on their overall HRQoL, as measured by the EQ VAS. Studies using the EQ-5D-3L have demonstrated a good relationship between these. They have consistently found that coefficients on the levels and dimensions of the EQ-5D-3L health state profile are in the correct direction and follow the expected gradient between levels, such that the coefficients on level 3 are greater than those on level 2 (Jelsma and Ferguson 2004; Whynes 2008, 2013; Feng et al. 2014).

Table 3.4 shows an example from the PROMs hip data used earlier.

Amongst possible interpretations of these results, it is notable that Anxiety & Depression has the biggest impact on the EQ VAS scores and Pain & Discomfort the smallest. Although level 2 Mobility has an impact similar to that of level 2 Self-care, level 3 has a much greater impact, perhaps reflecting the extreme nature of the EQ-5D-3L level 3 descriptor for Mobility ('confined to bed'). Similarly, although level 2 Usual Activities has a much lower impact than level 2 Self-care, the level 3 coefficients for these two dimensions are similar.

It is important to note that the coefficients that will be obtained are specific to the characteristics of the population from which the data are collected. For patient

Table 3.4 regression analysis of EQ VAS score against EQ-5D levels for hip replacement patients before surgery, English NHS 2010–11

	Coefficient	Standard Error
Mobility level 2	−5.64	0.472
Mobility level 3	−14.9	1.85
Self-care level 2	−5.20	0.234
Self-care level 3	−8.25	1.12
Usual activities level 2	−2.99	0.462
Usual activities level 3	−7.76	0.537
Pain & Discomfort level 2	−0.131	0.728
Pain & Discomfort level 3	−5.04	0.743
Anxiety & Depression level 2	−8.61	0.233
Anxiety & Depression level 3	−16.3	0.536
Intercept	83.2	0.814

Number of observations = 34 446
$R^2 = 0.166$, adjusted $R^2 = 0.166$, F = 686, p < 0.001
All coefficients significantly different from 0 at the 0.001 level

data, the evidence is that the profile coefficients may differ according to the type of condition that the patient has. Moreover, other variables, including age and sex, may impact not only on the EQ VAS scores directly but also on the profile coefficients, via interaction effects. Such analyses add further to understanding the impact of different patient characteristics and conditions on HRQoL. An additional implication is that simple comparisons between the coefficients obtained from this analysis and those obtained by modelling valuation data should be avoided.

As a direct illustration of this, Fig. 3.3, which has been generated from a vast amount of EQ-5D data held by the EuroQol Group office in Rotterdam, shows that there is a sharply declining EQ VAS by age for those whose self-reported profile contains at least some problems (Oppe 2013). As age increases, the number and severity of problems reported increase and the EQ VAS decreases. But the EQ VAS declines with age even among patients reporting no problems on any EQ-5D dimension.

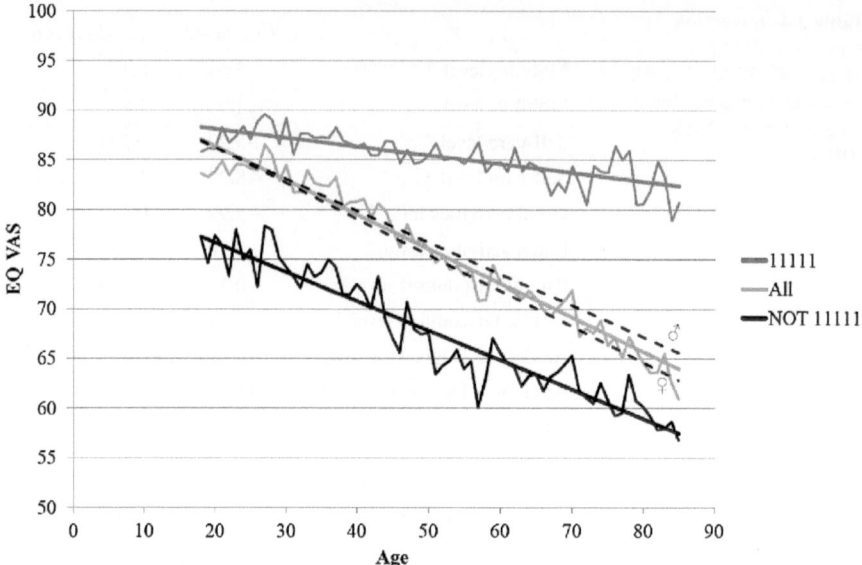

Fig. 3.3 The relationship between age and EQ VAS for those with no problems in any EQ-5D dimension and those with problems in at least one dimension (The straight lines are based on linear models for all data, no problems on EQ-5D (11111) and problems in at least one dimension (NOT 11111). The dashed straight lines represent separate linear models for men (♂) and women (♀) for all data. The other lines depict observed mean scores for corresponding groups.)

References

Devlin N, Parkin D, Browne J (2010) Patient Reported Outcomes in the NHS: new methods for analysing and reporting EQ-5D data. Health Econ 19(8):886–905

Devlin N, Lorgelly P, Herdman M (2019) Can we really compare and aggregate PRO data between people and settings? Implications for clinical trials and HTA. OHE Research Paper. www.ohe.org/publications/can-we-really-compare-and-aggregate-pro-data-between-peo ple-and-settings-implications

Feng Y, Parkin D, Devlin NJ (2014) Assessing the performance of the EQ VAS in the NHS PROMs Programme. Qual Life Res 23(3):977–989

Jelsma J, Ferguson G (2004) The determinants of self-reported health-related quality of life in a culturally and socially diverse South African community. Bull World Health Organ 82(3):206–212

Oppe M (2013) Mathematical approaches in economic evaluations: applying techniques from different disciplines. Erasmus University Rotterdam

Parkin D, Rice N, Jacoby A, Doughty J (2004) Use of a visual analogue scale in a daily patient diary: modelling cross-sectional time series data on health-related quality of life. Soc Sci Med 59(2):351–360

Whynes DK (2008) Correspondence between EQ-5D health state classifications and EQ VAS scores. Health Qual Life Outcomes 6:94

Whynes DK (2013) Does the correspondence between EQ-5D health state description and VAS score vary by medical condition? Health Qual Life Outcomes 11:155

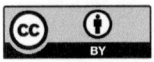

Chapter 4
Analysis of EQ-5D Values

The aims of this chapter are

- to introduce the properties and use of value sets;
- to highlight points to consider when choosing which value set to use;
- to provide guidance on statistical analysis of EQ-5D values, including descriptive statistics and inference; variance and heteroskedasticity; clustering; and regression methods; and
- to highlight the importance of conducting sensitivity analysis.

4.1 Value Sets and Their Properties

Despite the potential richness of the EQ-5D descriptive system demonstrated in the previous chapters, the instrument was originally developed as a measure of health status that could serve as the basis for summarising and comparing health outcomes (Williams 2005). In particular, it was designed to be a brief generic measure that would lend itself for the purpose of assigning a single summary value to each possible health profile (hereafter: 'EQ-5D values' or 'values'). The values, presented in country-specific value sets, are a major feature of the EQ-5D instrument, facilitating the calculation of quality-adjusted life years (QALYs) that are used to inform economic evaluations of health care interventions or policies on health.[1]

It is important to note that these values are a special case, based on people's strength of preference for different health profiles, of an index that generates a single summary number. Such indices in general (other than *values*), for example based on clinically-defined need, may be used for other purposes and, as we discuss below, it

---

[1] Note that it is beyond the scope of this book to offer guidance on how to conduct cost-effectiveness or cost-utility analysis. There are other resources providing detailed guidance on this, such as Drummond et al. (2015) and Sanders et al. (2016).

© The Author(s) 2020
N. Devlin et al., *Methods for Analysing and Reporting EQ-5D Data*,
https://doi.org/10.1007/978-3-030-47622-9_4

should not be assumed that using value sets is appropriate for any of those purposes.[2] Other possible uses of indices more broadly defined are to summarise EQ-5D profiles for statistical analysis, describing the health of a population, comparing population health (between regions, populations, or over time), describing severity of illness, and assessing population or patient priorities for treatment (Devlin and Parkin 2006). A relatively newly developed use is in routine outcomes measurement, to assess the performance of healthcare, for use as a hospital performance indicator (used to help patients choose which hospital to be referred to), and for use in measuring the productivity and performance of a healthcare system (Appleby et al. 2015).

A value set consists of weights that can convert each EQ-5D health profile into a value on a scale anchored at 1 (meaning full health) and 0 (meaning a state as bad as being dead). The scale allows negative values to be assigned to health states that are considered worse than dead. The values can be calculated by applying a formula that attaches a weight to each level in each dimension. In some cases, the formula allows for the possibility that combinations of problems might also affect preferences, via interaction effects.

The EQ-5D-3L describes 243 unique health profiles (3^5), whereas the EQ-5D-5L describes 3,125 possible unique health profiles (5^5). Most of the EQ-5D value sets have been obtained using stated preference data elicited from representative samples of the general public, thereby ensuring that they represent the societal perspective. The normative argument for using so-called "social" value sets is that for resource allocation purposes in publicly-or collectively-funded health care, the valuation of health states should reflect the preferences of the relevant general public (Weinstein et al. 1996; Sanders et al. 2016), since it is the general public who are ultimately funding health care and are the users of the health care system (Dolan 1997).

Value sets are commonly produced by valuing a selection of EQ-5D states and, by using econometric techniques, to extrapolate over the full set of health states. For the EQ-5D-3L, a subset of health states to be used in a valuation study was decided by the Group in 1990 (Rabin et al. 2007) along with a preferred method for obtaining the values, using a visual analogue scale (VAS) approach. For various reasons however, subsequent valuation studies have not always adhered to the standard approach, since these studies were often the result of locally led research initiatives. Apart from the choice of the health state design (i.e. deciding on the subset of states to be valued), studies differed in other ways, such as the valuation method and the (interviewer) protocol used, the number of respondents included, exclusion criteria for valuation responses, and modelling choices in arriving at a final value set. When the EQ-5D-5L was introduced, the EuroQol Group decided to return to having a more standardized approach by developing the EuroQol Valuation Technology platform (EQ-VT) (Oppe et al. 2014). Apart from standardization in terms of health state design, valuation methodology, and a computer-assisted personal interview mode of administration, a strict protocol of interviewer training and quality assurance during the entirety of the data collection process was developed and implemented (Ramos-Goñi et al. 2017a).

---

[2]However, we will only be discussing value sets in this chapter, not any other possible indices.

Values derived for EQ-5D have been based on various stated preference valuation techniques, such as the standard gamble (SG), time trade-off (TTO), VAS, person trade-off or rank-based techniques such as paired comparison, best-worse scaling and discrete choice methods. Since the first publication in 1997 (Dolan 1997), EQ-5D-3L value sets have been derived and published for many countries (www.eur oqol.org). EQ-5D-5L valuation studies have been conducted from 2012 onwards, and the published value sets are listed on the EuroQol website at www.euroqol.org. EQ-5D-3L value sets were mainly based on TTO and VAS valuation methodology, although other techniques have also been used (Craig et al. 2009; Bansback et al. 2012). For the valuation of EQ-5D-5L, the EuroQol Group decided to explore the use of rank-based valuation methods to gain additional information (Devlin and Krabbe 2013). The current EQ-VT protocol for the valuation of EQ-5D-5L health states uses composite TTO and discrete choice valuation methodology (Oppe et al. 2014). There has been much discussion about the theoretical and empirical properties of the different valuation methods. In the health economics literature choice-based methods such as SG and TTO are often argued to have a more solid basis in economic theory than a rating approach such as VAS (Brazier et al. 1999; Drummond et al. 2015)— although for an alternative view see Parkin and Devlin (2006)–whereas discrete choice methodology is rooted in mathematical psychology and was further developed into random utility theory (McFadden 1974).

The EQ-5D-5L descriptive system was published before valuation studies were carried out and the subsequent publication of value sets derived from them. As an interim measure, the EuroQol Group coordinated a study that administered both the 3-level and 5-level versions of the EQ-5D to develop a mapping[3] function between the EQ-5D-3L value sets and the EQ-5D-5L descriptive system, resulting in (interim) value sets for the EQ-5D-5L (van Hout et al. 2012). 3,691 respondents completed both the 3L and 5L across 6 countries: Denmark, England, Italy, the Netherlands, Poland and Scotland. Different subgroups were targeted, and in most countries, a screening protocol was implemented to ensure that a broad spectrum of levels of health would be captured across the dimensions of EQ-5D for both the 5L and 3L descriptive systems.

Table 4.1a, b show two existing value sets with examples how to calculate the values for a certain health profile.

Finally, an important consideration is that attaching values to descriptive data introduces an exogenous source of variance, which can bias statistical inference (Parkin et al. 2010; Wilke et al. 2010). This is a special problem for applications where people's preferences are not directly relevant and is a key reason why it should not be assumed that values provide a suitable index for non-economics applications. Conclusions about whether there are statistically significant differences in, for example, the health of 2 regions, or health over time, or between 2 arms of a clinical trial, may be influenced by which value set is used. Furthermore, note that there is no such thing as a neutral value set or index; any weighting of EQ-5D profile data will influence the results, including the equally weighted Level Sum Score

---

[3] For further information on mapping, see Sect. 5.2.

Table 4.1 **a** An example of applying the EQ-5D-3L value set for the United Kingdom (UK) to calculate EQ-5D values. **b** An example of applying the English EQ-5D-5L value set to calculate EQ-5D values

	Central estimate	Value for health profile 21232
Constant	1.000	1.000
At least one 2 or 3	0.081	0.081
At least one 3 (N3)	0.269	0.269
Mobility		
Some problems	0.069	0.069
Confined to bed	0.314	
Self-care		
Some problems	0.104	
Unable to	0.214	
Usual activities		
Some problems	0.036	0.036
Unable to	0.094	
Pain/discomfort		
Moderate	0.123	
Extreme	0.386	0.386
Anxiety/depression		
Moderate	0.071	0.071
Extreme	0.236	
The value for health state 21232	$1-(0.081 + 0.269 + 0.069 + 0.036 + 0.386 + 0.071) = 0.088$	
	Central estimate	Value for health profile 23245
Constant	1.000	1.000
Mobility		
Slight problems	0.058	0.058
Moderate problems	0.076	
Severe problems	0.207	
Unable to	0.274	
Self-care		
Slight problems	0.050	
Moderate problems	0.080	0.080
Severe problems	0.164	
Unable to	0.203	
Usual activities		
Slight problems	0.050	0.050
Moderate problems	0.063	
Severe problems	0.162	

(continued)

Table 4.1 (continued)

	Central estimate	Value for health profile 23245
Unable to	0.184	
Pain/discomfort		
Slight	0.063	
Moderate	0.084	
Severe	0.276	0.276
Extreme	0.335	
Anxiety/depression		
Slight	0.078	
Moderate	0.104	
Severe	0.285	
Extreme	0.289	0.289
The value for health state 23245	$1-(0.058 + 0.080 + 0.050 + 0.276 + 0.289) = 0.247$	

index described in Chap. 2. This is not specific to the EQ-5D, applying equally to the scoring systems of other health measures, both generic and condition specific, including measures that simply sum ranked responses. For economic evaluation, the issue is rather different, because the exogenous influence of people's preferences is a desired feature when taking a societal perspective.

4.2   Positive and Normative Considerations in Choice of Value Set

In recent decades, a large number of EQ-5D value sets have been published, using a multitude of approaches and valuation techniques, with applications in various fields. Users of EQ-5D often question what the appropriate value set is for their particular use. The aim of this section is to provide advice on this question, largely following the earlier "Guidance to users of EQ-5D value sets" which was published as Chapter 4 of the EuroQol Group Monographs Volume 2: EQ-5D value sets: Inventory, comparative review and user guide (Devlin and Parkin 2007).

An obvious advantage of using a summary value to represent a health profile is that it simplifies statistical analysis. But since all value sets embody preferences about the relative importance of each level of each dimension, it is not possible to offer generalised guidance about which value set to use if the objective is to summarise profiles for descriptive or inferential statistical analysis. If there is not a clear purpose for using a summary value (especially based on social values), but rather an aim to provide information, it may be better if no value is used, but to report the descriptive information as described in previous chapters. This also applies to describing the health of a population or patient group, or for comparing population health.

One of the most common uses of EQ-5D values remains in economic evaluation, with applications in cost-per-QALY/cost-effectiveness analysis (CEA) or cost-utility analysis (CUA). In CUA, the value set will be used to calculate QALYs, and the weights in the value set should represent "values", meaning that the health profiles described by the instrument should be weighed by the *value* of the health profile. To arrive at QALYs, the values should be anchored at 0 (corresponding to being dead or as bad as being dead), and 1, representing full health. A further requirement, although not essential for all cost-effectiveness analyses, is that the value set should be based on the societal perspective.

Often, economic evaluation is performed to provide evidence for a formal decision-making process. National health technology assessment bodies across the world routinely use economic evaluations to make decisions and recommendations about health care services. At the time of writing the EQ-5D is the preferred (or one of the preferred) health outcome measures recommended by pharmaceutical reimbursement authorities in at least 29 countries, including countries in Europe, North America, South America, Asia and Australia (Kennedy-Martin et al. 2020). When a value set needs to be selected to perform such an evaluation, the first consideration is pragmatic: does the relevant decision maker specify any requirements or preferences regarding which value set should be used? If recommendations will be made to more than one country on the basis of the evaluation's results, for example when performed alongside a multi-country clinical trial, the value set relevant to each separate country should be applied to the effectiveness data and reported to the decision makers in each separate country.

In the absence of specific requirements or guidelines from decision makers, analysts are left to make their own choices, for which broadly there are three main considerations to take into account: relevance to the decision-making context; empirical characteristics of the valuation study and modelling techniques; and the theoretical properties of the valuation methods.

Relevance to the decision-making context entails whether the values reflect the geographical and economic context in which resource allocation decisions are made, and whose values are considered to be relevant in the decision-making process. As mentioned in Sect. 4.1, there is a strong normative argument to opt for social valuations in economic evaluations informing decisions about collectively-funded health care. An alternative would be to use patients' values, because the preferences of patients who are actually experiencing the health states would be more well-informed than values generated from the general public being asked to imagine health states that may be hypothetical to them. Differences between patients' values and social values are widely observed (Zethraeus and Johannesson 1999; de Wit et al. 2000; Brazier et al. 2005; Ogorevc et al. 2019). Since the value set arguably should reflect the preferences of the potential recipients of healthcare, local (i.e. country-specific) value sets should be used when available. For a country for which no value set has been published and no local guidelines are available, practical aspects might be taken into consideration, such as considering a value set of a country that is most similar in terms of e.g. demographics, geography, language, infrastructure, or health care system. Finally, the time period in which the valuation study has been performed is relevant. The UK EQ-5D-3L value set is still being used extensively at the time of writing, but the data collection for the valuation study dates back to 1993, while the UK has gone through many demographic and economic changes since then which might impact on preferences.

Empirical characteristics should be considered when choosing a value set. It is recommended that users study those characteristics before choosing a value set, looking at e.g. the response rate of the valuation study, whether the sample was representative of the general public, which valuation method was used, whether the health state design was appropriate, which mode of administration was used, the 'quality' of the data (were there many missing values, inconsistencies, low values for very mild health states or vice versa), were the econometric modelling techniques sound and appropriate, was the choice of the final model appropriate? These questions largely apply to EQ-5D-3L, since with the introduction of the EQ-VT platform for the valuation of EQ-5D-5L, many potential issues have been resolved by a high level of standardization and rigorous interviewer training and quality assurance.

The theoretical properties of the underlying valuation methods have been a controversial issue for decades. As mentioned in Sect. 4.1, so-called 'choice-based' methods such as SG and TTO have been preferred over a rating approach such as VAS. For the EQ-5D-3L, mainly VAS and TTO value sets are available. TTO based value sets have generally been preferred for purposes of economic evaluation, although it has been suggested that VAS value sets may be used for non-economics studies (Kind 2003). The EQ-VT protocol for EQ-5D-5L valuation studies uses composite TTO and discrete choice valuation techniques, offering the possibility to model a composite TTO based value set, or a value set based on a hybrid model combining composite TTO and discrete choice data (Feng et al. 2018; Ramos-Goñi et al. 2017b).

Based on the criteria discussed above, there may not be a single 'best' value set for any given application. Therefore, it is recommended to perform sensitivity analysis using other suitable value sets, to assess the impact of the choice of value set on results and conclusions. As mentioned above, many countries do not have a value set of their own and therefore have to use 'foreign' values; Parkin et al. (2010) showed that in a simulated economic evaluation experiment, whether or not an intervention is seen as effective in such a country might depend on which other country's value set it chooses. This stresses the relevance of which value set one chooses, and the importance of performing sensitivity analysis (see Sect. 4.8).

The value sets that are used in economic evaluation have a clear theoretical rationale that is the foundation for the values, the way that they are derived, and their meaning. As mentioned above, this rationale might not be relevant for other uses. The values used in economic evaluation are explicitly regarded as 'utilities', with a very specific definition attached to them. There is a clear meaning for the values 1 and 0 and for negative values. As mentioned above, a recognized stated preference technique such as TTO is often recommended to derive the values. Finally, there is a justification for the use of the general population as a source of EQ-5D values. The values should be used in other applications only if the same theoretical rationale also applies.

Figure 4.1 provides an overview of the considerations that should determine your choice between the EQ-5D value sets. Choosing a value set is not simple, since many factors are involved, such as the specific nature of the research application, the sort of decisions it informs, and the context in which the evidence from your research will be used. In longitudinal studies, the same value set should be applied throughout the study. When the research aim is to make comparisons across respondents from

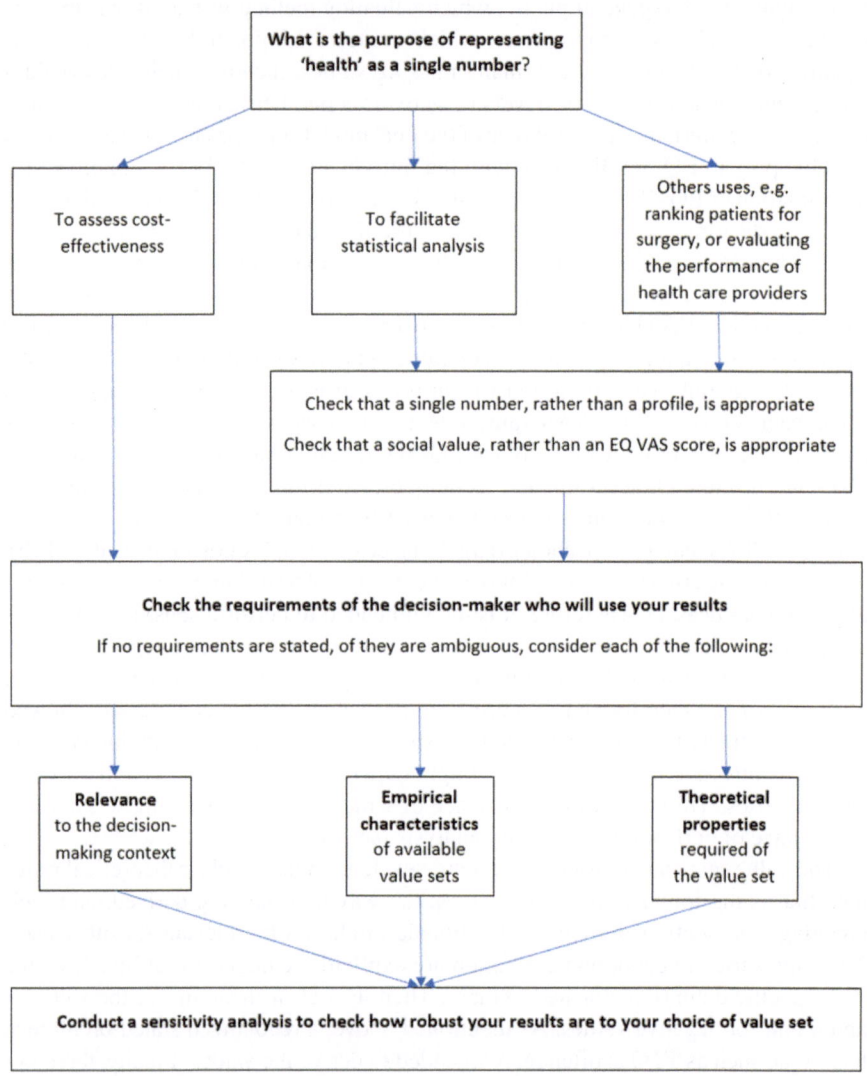

Fig. 4.1 Guidance on which EQ-5D value set to use

different countries in a multinational cross-sectional study (rather than comparing value set characteristics) it will also be helpful to use a common value set if one is available, otherwise differences in country preferences would be added to the differences between respondents' health status. An example is the European VAS value set (Greiner et al. 2003).

4.3 Simple Descriptive Statistics and Inference

EQ-5D values can be presented in much the same way as EQ VAS data. Since the valuation methods underlying the values are meant to provide a scale with cardinal properties, for exploratory data analysis you can present a measure of central tendency (e.g. a mean or median), a spread (i.e. a measure of dispersion such as the standard deviation) and a shape (e.g. skewness, mode, or kurtosis). If the data is skewed, as is often the case with EQ-5D value data for general populations or mildly diseased patients, the median value could be used as measure of central tendency. As measure of dispersion one can also add minimums, maximums, and the inter quartile range (IQR) which is the difference between the 75th and 25th percentiles. If you are interested in the precision of the mean, you can use the standard error of the mean and a 95% confidence interval. Similar to EQ VAS data, a t-test can be used for comparing differences between means of different populations (or the same population over time). When you want to compare more than 2 groups, an Analysis of variance (ANOVA) can be used. The following tables and figures contain 2 examples of how to present EQ-5D value results. Table 4.2 and Fig. 4.2 present the results from a study

Table 4.2 EQ-5D values before and after treatment

EQ-5D value	Before treatment	After treatment
Mean	0.567	0.727
Standard error	0.017	0.015
Median	0.60	0.810
Standard deviation	0.273	0.244
25th	0.331	0.606
75th	0.796	0.892
Kurtosis	2.96	5.18
Skewness	−0.734	−1.59
Minimum	−0.429	−0.349
Maximum	1	1
Range	1.429	1.349
Observations	251	249
Missing values (percent)	4 (1.6%)	3 (1.6%)

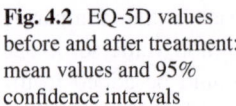

Fig. 4.2 EQ-5D values before and after treatment: mean values and 95% confidence intervals

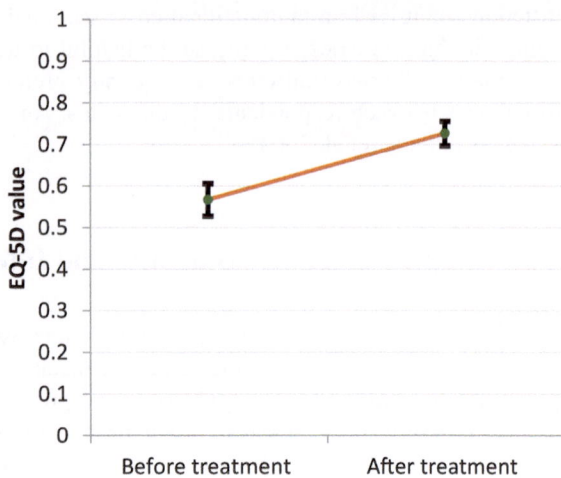

where the effect of a treatment on health status is investigated (the tables and figures are based on hypothetical data and for illustration purposes only).

Table 4.3 and Fig. 4.3 show results for a patient population and 3 sub-groups.

Below there are two more examples on how to report descriptive statistics for EQ-5D values. Table 4.4 shows a comprehensive overview of EQ-5D-3L population norm values for the United States (US), stratified by age and sex and also including total values. The precision of the estimate of the mean is indicated by the standard error. The median (50th percentile) is included, being relevant in general population samples that tend to be skewed towards full health, and a measure of dispersion is represented by the interquartile range (75th percentile–25th percentile).

An illustrative way to present longitudinal values from different populations is shown in Fig. 4.4 by a scatter plot for the experimental and comparator arms in an intervention design. One can simply track the value means for both patient groups over time, indicating the new treatment causes a more severe drop in health initially but also displays a quicker recovery and finally leads to a higher level of health than the comparator treatment.

Table 4.3 EQ-5D values for the total patient population and the 3 subgroups

EQ-5D value	All patients	Subgroup 1	Subgroup 2	Subgroup 3
Mean	0.660	0.450	0.550	0.900
Standard error	0.010	0.013	0.015	0.010
Median	0.550	0.400	0.550	0.950
25th	0.500	0.300	0.500	0.800
75th	0.700	0.500	0.600	1.000
N	300	100	75	125

Fig. 4.3 Mean EQ-5D values and 95% confidence intervals for the total patient population and 3 subgroups

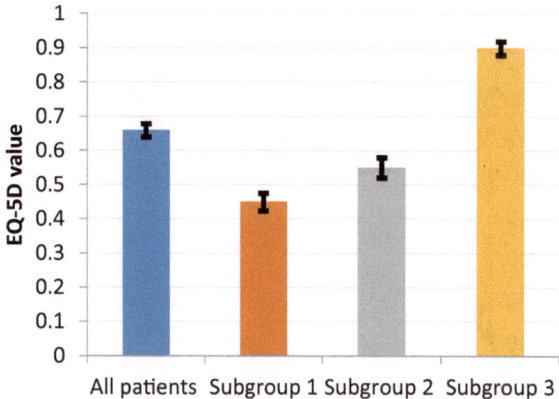

Table 4.4 General population EQ-5D-3L norm values for a representative sample of the US (Szende et al. 2014, Springer open access)

EQ-5D value		Age							
(TTO value set)		18–24	25–34	35–44	45–54	55–64	65–74	75+	Total
Total	Mean	0.925	0.912	0.888	0.855	0.827	0.813	0.754	0.866
	Standard error	0.002	0.002	0.002	0.002	0.003	0.003	0.004	0.001
	25th Percentile	0.83	0.83	0.83	0.80	0.78	0.78	0.71	0.80
	50th Percentile (median)	1.00	1.00	1.00	0.83	0.83	0.83	0.80	0.84
	75th Percentile	1.00	1.00	1.00	1.00	1.00	1.00	0.83	1.00
Males	Mean	0.935	0.921	0.900	0.864	0.842	0.825	0.773	0.880
	Standard error	0.003	0.003	0.003	0.003	0.004	0.005	0.007	0.001
	25th Percentile	0.84	0.83	0.83	0.81	0.80	0.78	0.71	0.82
	50th Percentile (median)	1.00	1.00	1.00	0.84	0.83	0.83	0.81	1.00
	75th Percentile	1.00	1.00	1.00	1.00	1.00	1.00	0.84	1.00
Females	Mean	0.914	0.904	0.877	0.846	0.812	0.803	0.741	0.854
	Standard error	0.003	0.003	0.003	0.003	0.004	0.005	0.005	0.001
	25th Percentile	0.83	0.83	0.81	0.80	0.78	0.77	0.71	0.80
	50th Percentile (median)	1.00	1.00	0.84	0.83	0.83	0.82	0.78	0.84
	75th Percentile	1.00	1.00	1.00	1.00	1.00	0.86	0.83	1.00

It is important to note that EQ-5D values are often not symmetrically distributed, and tend to be divided into multiple groups (clusters), which might mean that standard statistics such as means and standard deviations are harder to interpret. This will be discussed in more detail in Sects. 4.4 and 4.6.

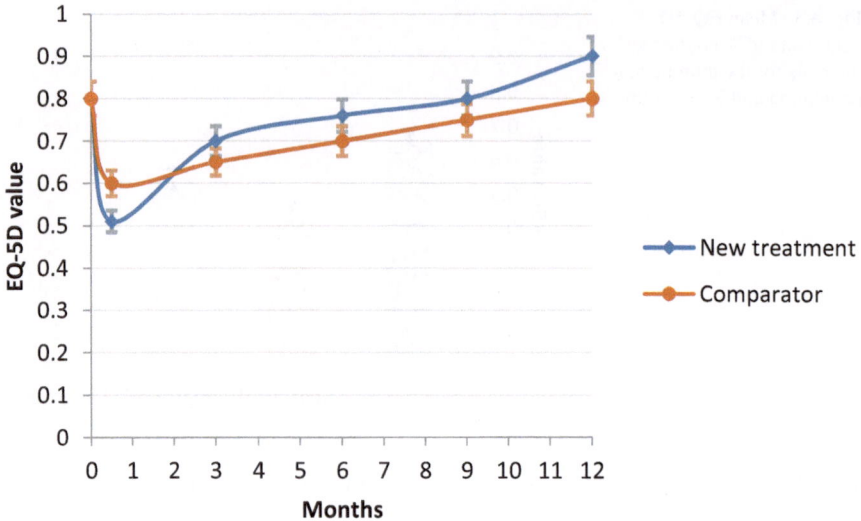

Fig. 4.4 Example of presentation of longitudinal EQ-5D values (hypothetical data with smoothed lines and confidence intervals)

EQ-5D values are often used to calculate QALYs, for use in CUA. Although QALYs are commonly used in an evaluative context, for example when comparing two or more health programmes. An example is shown here to calculate QALYs for descriptive purposes, e.g. for a single individual. In the standard QALY model, values are simply multiplied by the time period for the corresponding health state, and when different health states occur over time, these are added, as shown in Fig. 4.5, where two health states in suboptimal health occur with values ('utilities') of 0.4 and 0.8 after which health gradually improves after the initial event.

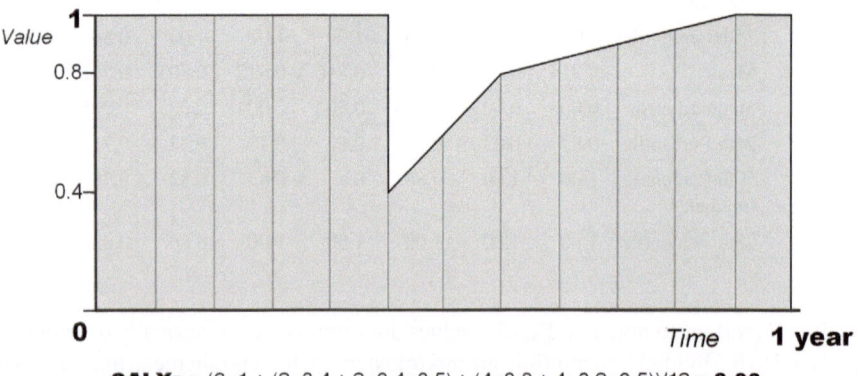

$$\textbf{QALYs} = (6 \times 1 + (2 \times 0.4 + 2 \times 0.4 \times 0.5) + (4 \times 0.8 + 4 \times 0.2 \times 0.5))/12 = \textbf{0.90}$$

Fig. 4.5 QALY calculation of an event-like condition with a recovery period

4.4   Examining the Distribution of the EQ-5D Values

Examining EQ-5D value distributions can be done in a graphical as well as in a numerical manner. First, we present graphical ways of exploring distributions. Distributions of EQ-5D values often show gaps and spikes or clusters of observations in certain parts of the scale. At the upper part of the scale there is often a gap which can be quite substantial, especially in EQ-5D-3L value distributions. This gap is caused by the ceiling often present in EQ-5D data and the intercept in the value function. In general population samples, but also in mildly or moderately diseased samples, often a relatively large proportion of respondents score no problems on all five dimensions: the ceiling. A large ceiling will result in a skewed distribution. For many value sets, there is a relatively large constant (or intercept) in the value set, leading to a gap between full health and the second-best health state. In distributional terms this may result in at least two clusters in the distribution. Apart from this "upper gap", more gaps may appear in EQ-5D value distributions. Parkin et al. (2016) demonstrated that two or three clusters often occur in value distributions for EQ-5D-3L. The left panel in Fig. 4.6 shows an example with 3 clusters caused by the ceiling and the intercept (the upper gap) and a low and high cluster which are caused by differences between levels 2 and 3 value decrements being greater than those between levels 1 and 2, and also because of the so-called N3 term[4] used in the many EQ-5D-3L value sets, as shown by Parkin et al. The right panel in Fig. 4.6 shows a distribution of EQ-5D-5L in the same patient group, resulting in a much smoother distribution. Note that these data were derived from a single patient sample: these respondents scored both the EQ-5D-3L and EQ-5D-5L descriptive systems, and subsequently the corresponding value sets (UK for EQ-5D-3L and English for EQ-5D-5L) were applied to the health profile data.

There are several differences between value sets across countries, but overall it was shown that EQ-5D-5L distributions resulted in smoother and more natural

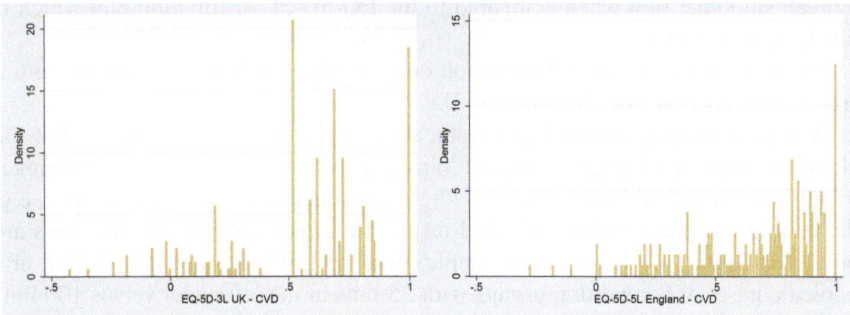

Fig. 4.6 Distribution of EQ-5D-3L and EQ-5D-5L values in a sample of cardiovascular disease (CVD) patients (N = 251)

---

[4]The N3 term results in an additional decrement of the value when at least one level 3 is present in the health profile.

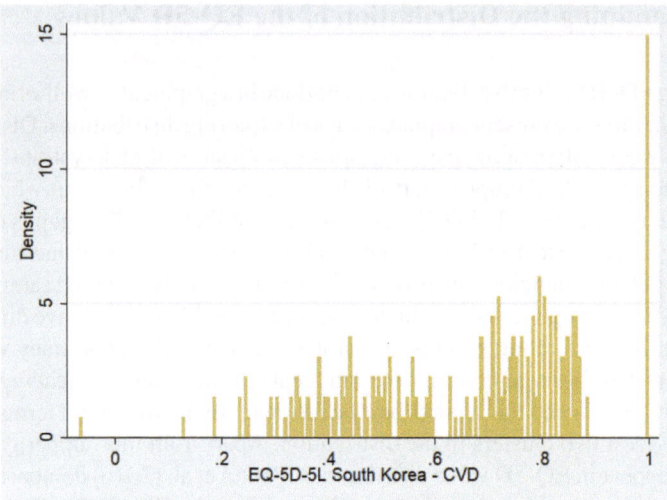

Fig. 4.7 Distribution of EQ-5D-5L values in a sample of cardiovascular disease patients (N = 251)

looking distributions than EQ-5D-3L (Janssen et al. 2018). Interestingly, an exception occurred for an EQ-5D-5L value set including a model term similar to N3. Here again three clusters appear in the distribution, as depicted in Fig. 4.7.

Sometimes histograms of distributions are not easy to assess, especially with large datasets in heterogeneous populations, e.g. showing a large spread of observations and perhaps spikes or clusters across the value scale. It becomes even more difficult when you want to compare two distributions in a single figure. In these cases, it might help to use a smoothing function such as the kernel density estimation. Figure 4.8 shows an example of an EQ-5D-3L and EQ-5D-5L kernel density plot in a large heterogeneous dataset. Note that also here the EQ-5D-5L distribution resulted in a much smoother plot when compared to the EQ-5D-3L distribution plot which is much more irregular.

When depicting a single distribution one can also combine a histogram with a smoothing function, such as shown in Fig. 4.9.

A final comment in regard to graphical presentation by histograms is that the choice of number of interval ranges ("bins", each bar represents 1 interval range) might influence the density in areas with a high concentration of observations, e.g. the ceiling (proportion of 11111) will result in a larger spike when more bins are opted for. Figure 4.10 shows an example for an EQ-5D-5L value distribution in a pooled dataset of 9 condition groups with 35 bins in the left panel versus 100 bins in the right panel.

Many EQ-5D-3L value set distributions will result in a distribution with clusters and gaps. These patterns in the distribution are considered to be undesirable as they can diminish the sensitivity and accuracy of the instrument (Janssen et al. 2018). Moreover, they can lead to estimation problems if distributions result in a

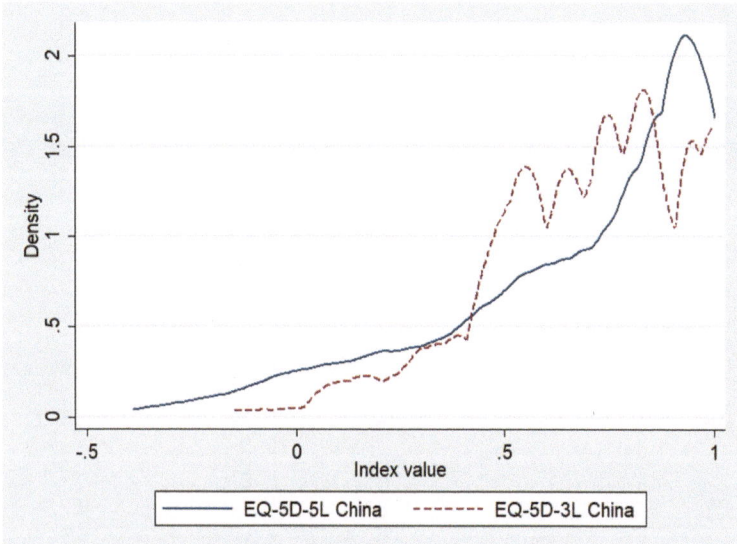

Fig. 4.8 Distribution of EQ-5D-3L and EQ-5D-5L values in a pooled dataset of 9 condition groups (N = 3,790)

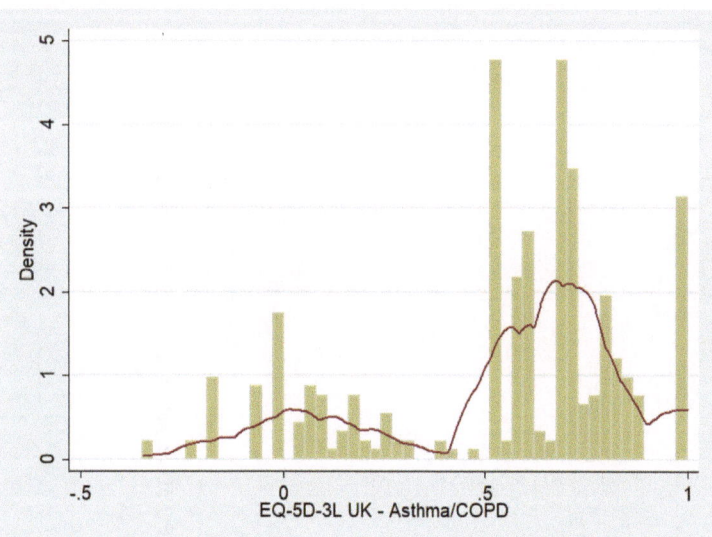

Fig. 4.9 Distribution of EQ-5D-3L values in a sample of Asthma/COPD patients (N = 342)

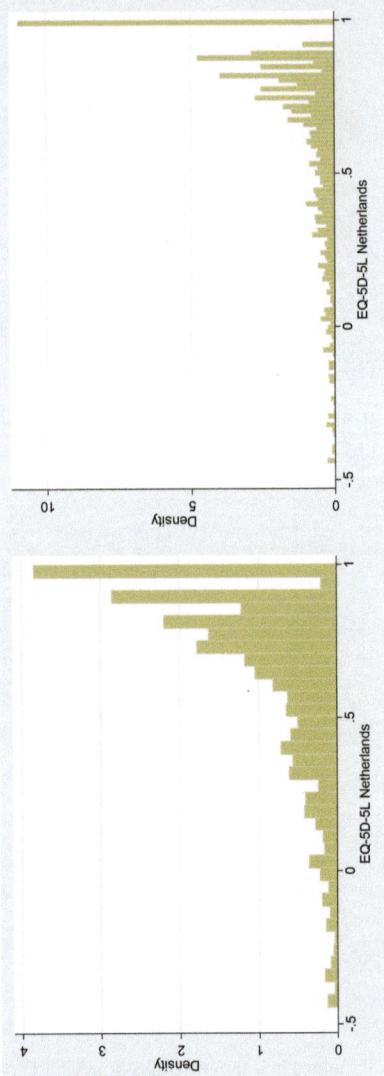

Fig. 4.10 Distribution of EQ-5D-5L values applying 35 versus 100 bins

violation of homoscedasticity[5] when the values are used as dependent variable in regression analysis. With the introduction of the EQ-5D-5L the clusters and gaps largely disappeared, although to a lesser extent they still might occur. An extreme example is shown in Fig. 4.7 where clusters were caused by the large intercept and the interaction term in the value function. For other EQ-5D-5L country-specific value sets clusters and gaps hardly occur. Overall the interim ('mapped') EQ-5D-5L value distributions tend to be more similar in shape to the EQ-5D-5L value set distributions, although the range is identical to the EQ-5D-3L distributions (Feng et al. 2019; Mulhern et al. 2018). In Sects. 4.6 and 4.7 guidance is provided on how to deal with a clustered data distribution.

A final remark can be made in regard to the terms bimodal and even trimodal that are often used to describe distributions with 2 or 3 clusters respectively. Parkin et al. (2016) point out that in regard to EQ-5D-3L data these terms are misleading, since the modes of the groups are not their most interesting feature. The groups do not always have a single local mode, and in practice these modes are never actually identified, reported, or analysed.

There are several numerical ways of assessing EQ-5D value distributions. A simple way is to report the proportion of the ceiling and the floor. More comprehensive methods are evenness measures such as the Shannon indices, or the Health State Density Index as described in Sect. 2.8. Note that the total number of unique *values* might be (almost) equal to the number of unique possible *health profiles*. In these cases, the resulting indices will be equal to or close to the indices applied to the profile data.

4.5 Variance and Heteroskedasticity

As described above, EQ-5D value data is often defined by some specific characteristics. By nature, the data are censored due to the upper bound at 1 (full health) and the lower bound for the most severe health profile (33333 in 3L and 55555 in 5L). Because 11111 describes full or "normal" health as indicated by having no problems across the five dimensions, there often is a ceiling present and the data distribution might be skewed. A consequence of these factors is that variances might vary across the value space, leading to heteroskedasticity. Heteroskedasticity refers to the situation where the variance of a variable is unequal across the range of values of a second variable that describes or predicts it. Figure 4.11 shows an example of observed values paired with self-reported EQ VAS ratings. Typically EQ-5D variances will be unequal across the scale, which is at least partly due to the censored nature of the value scale (e.g. the figure clearly shows reduced variance in the upper right corner of the Fig. 4.11).

A graphical way of depicting heteroskedasticity (or homoscedasticity) is by using a residual-versus-predictor plot, which is a scatter plot of residuals against the

---

[5]See also Sect. 4.6.

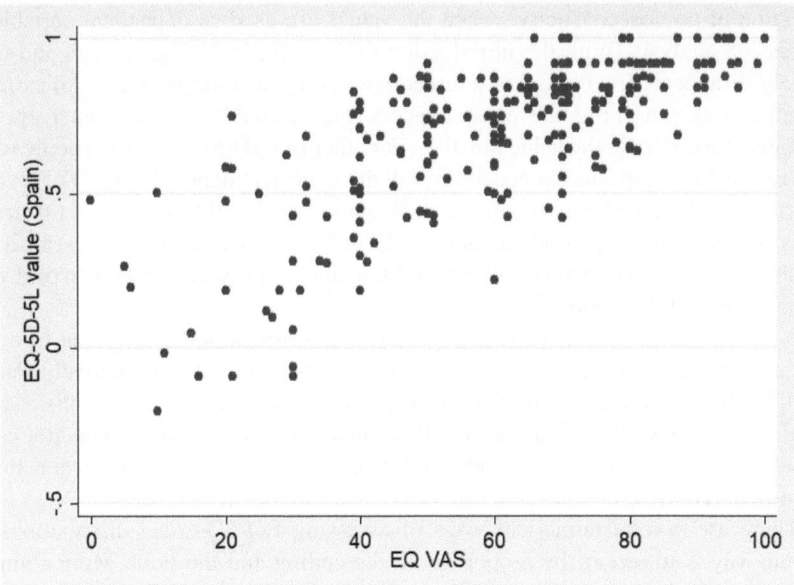

Fig. 4.11   EQ-5D-5L values (Spanish value set) plotted against EQ VAS for a sample of personality disorder patients (n = 384)

predicted values. One can easily detect if there are any patterns visible in the scatter plot. If there are no visible patterns or the plot shows roughly a rectangular shape, or both, the data are likely to be homoscedastic. Note that a pattern could be present in a residual-versus-predictor plot but the data could still be homoscedastic, in which case the data is likely to be biased. Figure 4.12 shows an example of a residual-versus-predictor plot for the same data used in Fig. 4.11. Clearly residuals are distributed unequally across the value scale which means that heteroskedasticity is present.

There have been many reported cases of heteroscedasticity in EQ-5D data. Section 4.7 provides further information on how to deal with heteroscedasticity in EQ-5D data.

4.6   Exploring Clusters in EQ-5D Value Distributions

As described in Sect. 4.4, EQ-5D value distributions often show clusters of obser-vations. Sometimes these can be clearly detected graphically as is the case for many EQ-5D-3L distributions. In other cases, one can use statistical methods to test for the presence of clusters. A distribution with multiple clusters might imply that there are actually multiple patient populations that should be analysed separately. The mean value might actually refer to a point on the value scale were there are hardly any observations, so perhaps a better way to inform about these data would be to report

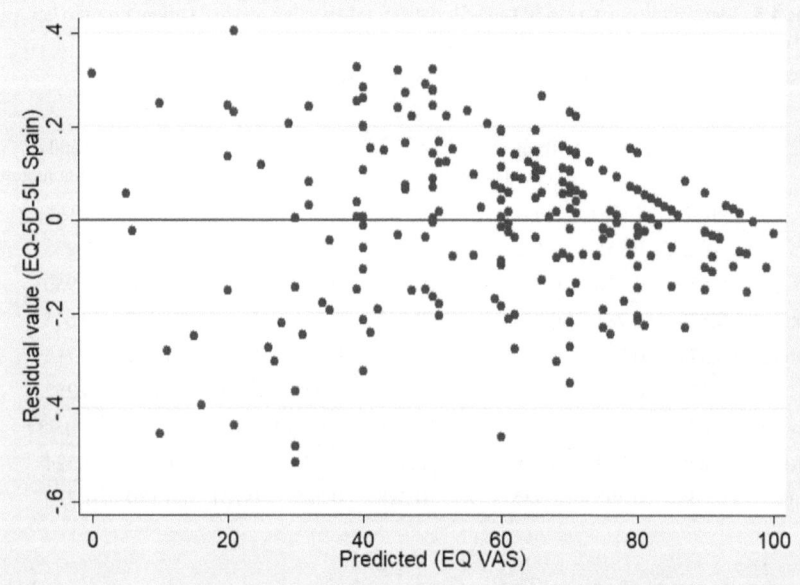

Fig. 4.12 Residual-versus-predictor plot of EQ-5D-5L residual values (Spanish value set) plotted against EQ VAS (ordinary least squares regression) in a sample of personality disorder patients (n = 384)

simple descriptive statistics such as the mean, median, mode, range and standard deviations for the clusters *separately*.

Parkin et al. (2016) and Feng et al. (2019) used statistical techniques to detect clusters, first by applying k-means clustering to demonstrate the presence of clusters in EQ-5D-3L and EQ-5D-5L distributions. The k-means cluster algorithm searches for the optimal partition in *k* clusters. There are many stopping rules available for determining the optimal number of clusters. Feng et al. identified the Calinski-Harabasz pseudo-F index as the most suitable stopping rule for EQ-5D value data. Before applying the k-means procedure, the number of clusters must be decided upon. Subsequently the stopping rule may be applied to determine the optimal number of clusters. For more detail see Feng et al. (2019). Table 4.5 shows an example of applying this method on the EQ-5D-5L value set for England in a large pooled dataset across 2 patient groups. There are different clusters apparent, with different mean values and different dispersion and shape statistics. Note that different clusters are found for the different patient groups, and also the optimal number of clusters varies over the different patient groups.

Although this approach can be used as a useful exploratory tool, it does involve arbitrary judgments. Therefore, a careful examination of the data and resulting cluster statistics is advised before making conclusions in regard to what the optimal clusters are, if any. Testing for clusters and identifying clusters can be useful before using the data for different applications, such as health technology assessment and health

Table 4.5 Identifying clusters in EQ-5D-5L data (English value set) in 2 patient groups (Feng et al. 2019)

Cluster	Musculoskeletal Patients			Specialist nursing patients				
	K = 2			K = 4				
	1	2	Total (unclustered)	1	2	3	4	Total (unclustered)
N	5051	14551	19602	253	571	916	1182	2922
Min	−0.285	0.555	−0.285	−0.285	0.246	0.535	0.770	0.285
Max	0.553	0.950	0.950	0.243	0.531	0.766	0.950	0.950
Mean	0.329	0.781	0.664	0.092	0.396	0.669	0.867	0.645
Median	0.374	0.795	0.732	0.119	0.399	0.674	0.864	0.715
SD	0.178	0.099	0.233	0.123	0.082	0.063	0.055	0.252
Skewness	−0.925	−0.297	−1.235	−0.920	−0.100	−0.353	−0.082	−0.982
Kurtosis	3.255	2.234	4.096	2.941	1.726	2.079	1.699	3.324
Range	0.838	0.395	1.235	0.528	0.285	0.231	0.180	1.235

care management processes. The statistical techniques one intends to use should take account of clustering, in order to ensure that inferences drawn from the results are not biased.

An exploratory potential use of cluster analysis is to provide a means of identifying distinct pre-and post-treatment patient groups, and to use that information to predict which patients might benefit the most from the treatment and for which the treatment is less successful.

4.7   Regression Analysis

Regression analysis is a commonly used statistical technique for analysing EQ-5D values, quantifying the influence on values of their underlying determinants, such as clinical and socioeconomic characteristics. Applying multivariate regression enables multivariate comparisons, similar to the analysis of EQ VAS scores, as described in Sect. 3.3. The main uses are within economic evaluation, where the interest is in the values generated by different health care interventions, and in mapping studies, where the interest is in the values attached to different health states.

In Table 4.6 an example is shown of applying regression techniques for economic modelling for a treatment for relapsed or refractory multiple myeloma (NICE 2017). EQ-5D-3L data (UK value set) resulting from a randomized controlled trial were modelled by regression analysis for use in CUA. A repeated measurement mixed model was used to predict EQ-5D-3L values based on three types of response, whether a patient was ≤3 months prior to death, hospitalizations, (treatment related) adverse events, and new primary malignancies. The occurrence of adverse events and

Table 4.6   Utility coefficients for parameters obtained using the EQ-5D-3L (UK value set)[a]

Parameter	Coefficient	Standard error	95% Confidence Limits	95% Confidence limits	Z	Pr > |Z|
Intercept	−1.245	0.038	−1.319	−1.170	−32.950	<0.001
PD	0.182	0.054	0.077	0.287	3.400	0.001
PR	0.122	0.056	0.012	0.232	2.180	0.029
SD	0.187	0.061	0.068	0.305	3.080	0.002
Hospitalisation	0.219	0.203	−0.178	0.617	1.080	0.279
Grade 3 or 4 TRAE	0.055	0.036	−0.016	0.127	1.52	0.13
New Primary Malignancy	0.713	0.052	0.611	0.815	13.70	<0.0001
EOL 0-3 months pre-death	0.378	0.081	0.219	0.537	4.65	<0.0001

Key: EOL, end of life; PD, progressed disease; PR, partial response; SD, stable disease; TRAE, treatment related adverse events

[a]EQ-5D-3L data were transposed into a utility decrement using "decrement = 1−utility". The decrements were used as dependent variables in the regression model with response status, hospitalisation, adverse events, new primary malignancy, whether a patient is within 3 months prior to death, treatment allocation and time as independent variables, with interactions between time and response status

hospitalisation were included as covariates. The model used a log link and a Gamma distribution. The results from this regression showed that new primary malignancies and whether a patient is ≤3 months prior to death had the largest effects on utility. Variables associated with response status also had a significant impact. The coefficients associated with adverse events and hospitalisations were not significant. The utility coefficients can be used for the calculation of QALYs for inclusion in a CUA model.

As we have seen in Sect. 4.4, EQ-5D data is characterized by its censored nature with bounds at full health and the worst health state. Moreover, for many country-specific EQ-5D value sets, there is a gap between full health and the second best health state. For EQ-5D-3L, there are often clusters present, which only occurs for certain country-specific value sets for EQ-5D-5L data. Given this specific nature of EQ-5D values, many different regression techniques have been applied.

Ordinary Least Squares (OLS) regression is the most commonly used regression technique. As always, it is necessary to test for violations of its underlying assumptions, although it is robust to small violations, especially in large samples. These include the assumption that the residuals are normally distributed[6] and homoscedastic, violations of which affect statistical testing of regression coefficients,

---

[6]Note that the data itself do not need to be normally distributed due to the Central Limit Theorem. The distribution of the means of non-normal distributions will still be normal as long as the samples are large enough, large being roughly above 30 (Norman and Streiner 2000, p. 28).

though not the estimates themselves. However, EQ-5D values data may be subject to clustering, which violates the assumption that all of the observations in the data are independent, and censoring, which could affect the consistency of the OLS estimator, generating estimates that may be biased.

Various statistical tests are available to verify which regression techniques are most suitable for a given dataset. Normality of residuals can be assessed by several formal tests, including skewness and kurtosis estimates, the Shapiro-Wilk test, or the Jarque-Bera test. When using EQ-5D data in regression analysis, it is recommended to test for heteroskedasticity, for which many formal tests are available, such as the Breusch-Pagan test or the White test. When comparing two or more groups one also has to take the possibility of unequal variances into account. Again, it is recommended to test for unequal variances, e.g. by using the F-test of equality of variances. Note that the assumption of homoscedasticity is related to the residuals and not the dependent and independent variables included in a regression itself. Graphical and numerical approaches as described in Sects. 4.4 and 4.6 can be applied to test for the presence of clusters. Based on these results, one can determine which regression technique is most suited for the analysis of interest.

Many regression modelling techniques are available to deal with the typical nature of EQ-5D value data, such as Tobit, censored least absolute deviation (CLAD) or other median models, two-part models, latent-class models, and limited dependent variable mixture models[7] (Austin 2002; Fu and Kattan 2006; Huang et al. 2008; Pullenayegum et al. 2010; Hernández Alava et al. 2012). These different models aim to deal with various characteristics of the data. Tobit and CLAD models can take account of the censored nature of EQ-5D data. Two-part models specifically take the ceiling effect and the upper gap into account. Pullenayegum et al. (2010) suggested that Tobit and CLAD models might lead to biased results and propose OLS coupled with robust standard errors or the nonparametric bootstrap as a simpler and more valid approach which corrects for heteroskedasticity. Hernández Alava et al. (2012) demonstrated that an adjusted limited dependent variable approach combined with a mixture model can also account for the typical nature of EQ-5D-3L data (censored, large upper gap, and clustering). Figure 4.13 shows how the various models relate to different distributions, and we can indeed see that the adjusted limited dependent variable mixture model might be a good fit for various EQ-5D-3L distributions. For EQ-5D-5L, less complex models might suffice.

The mixture model approach applied by Hernández Alava et al. can also be used to identify latent classes, which bears a resemblance to identifying clusters as described in Sect. 4.6. A latent class model might be applied in regression to account for the different classes or clusters.

We end this section by providing an example. An innovative technique to develop a "catalogue" of EQ-5D-3L values by applying regression techniques to a large representative population survey database collected in the US was introduced by Sullivan and Ghushchyan (2006). CLAD regression was used to estimate the marginal

---

[7]Note that Hernández Alava et al. (2012) use a wider term (limited dependent variable) for EQ-5D data being censored at 1.

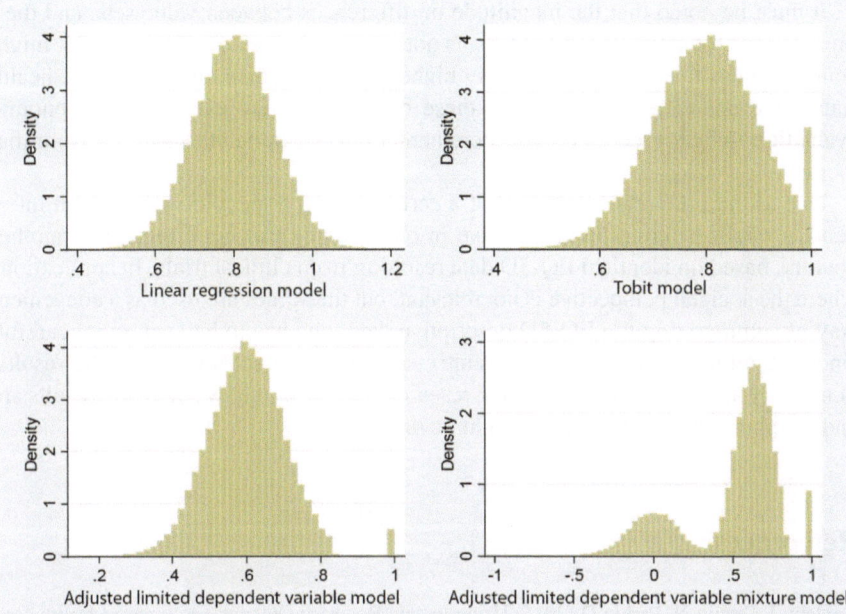

Fig. 4.13 Illustrative histograms of possible model distributions (Hernández Alava, copyright Value in Health)

disutility of conditions classified by International Classification of Diseases codes (Ninth Revision), controlling for age, comorbidity, gender, race, ethnicity, income, and education. The resulting list of EQ-5D-3L values could serve as an "off-the-shelf" catalogue that might be used by analysts to estimate QALYs in CUA.

4.8 Uncertainty and Sensitivity Analysis

As mentioned in Sect. 4.2, since there may not be a single 'best' value set for any given application, it is recommended to perform sensitivity analysis using other suitable value sets in order to assess the impact of the choice of value set on results and conclusions. Parkin et al. (2010) showed that the choice of value set might determine whether an intervention is seen as effective or not. Since many countries do not have a value set of their own, the choice of value set as well as performing sensitivity analysis, is very important. The analyst conducting CUA should treat the values in an economic evaluation as uncertain parameters which, just like other non-stochastic uncertain variables such as the discount rate, should be subject to sensitivity analysis, in order to improve confidence in the obtained results.

It must be noted that the magnitude of differences between value sets, and their implications for estimates of QALYs, is not always obvious. As one value set might contain values that are systematically higher (or lower) than another for the health states relevant to a given therapy, these differences may even out in economic evaluation, which focuses on the incremental change in health resulting from that therapy.

Due to the preference structure of a certain country-specific value set, an intervention might be considered effective in one country and not effective in another country, based on identical EQ-5D data resulting from clinical trials. In applications where the societal perspective is not relevant, but the values are used as a convenient way of summarizing the EQ-5D descriptive data, one has to be even more careful, since the influence on any given country-specific value set might bias the results. Sensitivity analysis will also give the researcher a sense of how stable the results are and whether robust conclusions might be drawn.

References

Appleby J, Devlin N, Parkin D (2015) Using Patient Reported Outcomes to improve health care. Wiley Blackwell

Austin PC (2002) A comparison of methods for analyzing health-related quality of life measures. Value Health 5:329–37

Bansback N, Brazier J, Tsuchiya A, Anis A (2012) Using a discrete choice experiment to estimate health state utility values. J Health Econ 31(1):306–318

Brazier J, Deverill M, Green C (1999) A review of the use of health status measures in economic evaluation. J Health Serv Res Policy 4(3):174–184

Brazier J, Akehurst, R, Brennan, A Dolan P, Claxton K, McCabe C, Sculpher M, Tsuchyia A (2005) Should patients have a greater role in valuing health states? Appl Health Econ Health Policy 4(4):201–208

Craig BM, Busschbach JJ, Salomon JA (2009) Keep it simple: ranking health states yields values similar to cardinal measurement approaches. J Clin Epidemiol 62(3):296–305

Devlin N, Parkin D (2007) Guidance to users of EQ-5D value sets. In: Szende A, Oppe M, Devlin N (eds) EQ-5D value sets: inventory, comparative review and user guide. Springer, Dordrecht, The Netherlands

de Wit GA, Busschbach JJ, de Charro FTH (2000) Sensitivity and perspective in the valuation of the health status: whose values count? Health Econ 9:109–126 www.euroqol.org, Accessed June 2nd 2019

Devlin NJ, Krabbe PF (2013) The development of new research methods for the valuation of EQ-5D-5L. Eur J Health Econ 14(Suppl 1):S1–S3

Dolan P (1997) Modeling valuations for EuroQol health states. Med Care 35(11):1095–1108

Drummond MF, Sculpher MJ, Claxton K, Stoddart GL, Torrance GW (2015) Methods for the economic evaluation of health care programmes, 4th edn. Oxford University Press, Oxford

Feng Y, Devlin N, Bateman A, Zamora B, Parkin D. (2019) Distribution of the EQ-5D-5L Profiles and Values in Three Patient Groups. Value Health 22(3):355–361

Feng Y, Devlin NJ, Shah KK, Mulhern B, van Hout B (2018) New methods for modelling EQ-5D-5L value sets: an application to English data. Health Econ 27(1):23–38

Fu AZ, Kattan MW (2006) Racial and ethnic differences in preference-based health status measure. Curr Med Res Opin 22(12):2439–2448

Greiner W, Weijnen T, Nieuwenhuizen M, Oppe S, Badia X, Busschbach J, Buxton M, Dolan P, Kind P, Krabbe P, Ohinmaa A, Parkin D, Roset M, Sintonen H, Tsuchiya A, de Charro F (2003) A single European currency for EQ-5D health states. results from a six-country study. Eur J Health Econ 4(3):222–31

Hernández Alava M, Wailoo AJ, Ara R (2012) Tails from the peak district: adjusted limited dependent variable mixture models of EQ-5D questionnaire health state utility values. Value Health 15(3):550–561

Huang IC, Frangakis C, Atkinson MJ et al (2008) Addressing ceiling effects in health status measures: a comparison of techniques applied to measures for people with HIV disease. Health Serv Res 43(1 Pt 1):327–339

Janssen MF, Bonsel GJ, Luo N (2018) Is EQ-5D-5L better than EQ-5D-3L? A head-to-head comparison of descriptive systems and value sets from seven countries. Pharmacoecononomics 36(6):675–697

Kennedy-Martin M, Slaap B, Herdman M, van Reenen M et al (2020) Which multi-attribute utility instruments are recommended for use in cost-utility analysis? A review of national health technology assessment (HTA) guidelines. Eur J Health Econ doi: 10.1007/s10198-020-01195-8 Online ahead of print

Kind P (2003) Guidelines for value sets in economic and non-economic studies using EQ-5D. In: Brooks R, Rabin R, de Charro F (eds) The measurement and valuation of health status using EQ-5D: a European perspective. Kluwer Academic Publisher, Dordrecht, pp 29–41

McFadden D (1974) Conditional logit analysis of qualitative choice behavior. In: Zarembka P (ed) Frontiers in Econometrics. Academic Press, New York

Mulhern B, Feng Y, Shah K, Janssen MF, Herdman M, van Hout B, Devlin N (2018) Comparing the UK EQ-5D-3L and English EQ-5D-5L value sets. Pharmacoecononomics 6(6):699–713

NICE 2017. https://www.nice.org.uk/guidance/ta505/documents/committee-papers

Norman GR, Streiner DL (2000) Biostatistics: the bare essentials, 2nd edn. BC Decker Incorporated, Hamilton

Ogorevc M, Murovec N, Fernandez NB, Rupel VP (2019) Questioning the differences between general public vs. patient based preferences towards EQ-5D-5L defined hypothetical health states. Health Policy 123(2):166–172

Oppe M, Devlin NJ, van Hout B, Krabbe PF, de Charro F (2014) A program of methodological research to arrive at the new international EQ-5D-5L valuation protocol. Value Health 17(4):445–453

Parkin D, Devlin N (2006) Is there a case for using visual analogue scale valuations in cost-utility analysis? Health Econ 15(7):653–664

Parkin D, Rice N, Devlin N (2010) Statistical analysis of EQ-5D profiles: does the use of value sets bias inference? Med Decis Making 30(5):556–565

Parkin D, Devlin N, Feng Y (2016) What determines the shape of an EQ-5D index distribution? Med Decision Making 36(8):941–951

Pullenayegum EM, Tarride J, Xie F, Goeree R, Gerstein HC, O'Reilly D (2010) Analysis of health utility data when some subjects attain the upper bound of 1: are Tobit and CLAD models appropriate? Value Health 13:487–494

Rabin R, de Charro F, Szende A (2007) Introduction. In: Szende A, Oppe M, Devlin N (eds) EQ-5D value sets: inventory, comparative review and user guide. Springer, Dordrecht, The Netherlands

Ramos-Goñi JM, Oppe M, Slaap B, Busschbach JJ, Stolk E (2017a) Quality control process for EQ-5D-5L valuation studies. Value Health 20(3):466–473

Ramos-Goñi JM, Pinto-Prades JL, Oppe M, Cabasés JM, Serrano-Aguilar P, Rivero-Arias O (2017b) Valuation and modeling of EQ-5D-5L health states using a hybrid approach. Med Care 55(7):e51–e58

Sanders GD, Neumann PJ, Basu A et al (2016) Recommendations for conduct, methodological practices, and reporting of cost-effectiveness analyses: second panel on cost-effectiveness in health and medicine. JAMA 316(10):1093–1103

Sullivan PW, Ghushchyan V (2006) Preference-based EQ-5D index scores for chronic conditions in the United States. Med Decis Making 26(4):410–420

Szende A, Janssen MF, Cabases J (2014) Self-reported population health: an international perspective based on EQ-5D. Springer, Dordrecht

van Hout B, Janssen MF, Feng Y et al (2012) Interim scoring for the EQ-5D-5L: mapping the EQ-5D-5L to EQ-5D-3L value sets. Value in Health 15:708–715

Weinstein MC, Siegel JE, Gold MR, Kamlet MS, Russell LB (1996) Recommendations of the Panel on Cost-Effectiveness in Health and Medicine. JAMA 276(15):1253–1258

Wilke CT, Pickard AS, Walton SM, Moock J, Kohlmann T, Lee TA (2010) Statistical implications of utility weighted and equally weighted HRQL measures: an empirical study. Health Econ 19(1):101–110

Williams A (2005) The EuroQol instrument. In: Kind P, Brooks R, Rabin R (eds) EQ-5D concepts and methods: a developmental history. Springer, Dordrecht

Zethraeus N, Johannesson M (1999) A comparison of patient and social tariff values derived from the time trade-off method. Health Econ 8:541–545

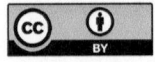

Chapter 5
Advanced Topics

This chapter provides guidance on a number of advanced topics, building on the content of earlier chapters. Our aims are

- to show how changes and differences in EQ-5D values and EQ VAS scores can be analysed;
- to discuss what a Minimally Important Difference (MID) means in the context of EQ-5D data and some of the challenges to the use of MIDs;
- to explain why case-mix adjustment of EQ-5D data is important in some contexts, and how that might be done; and
- to provide an overview of the use of mapping techniques to link other Patient Reported Outcome (PRO) data to the EQ-5D and EQ-5D values.

5.1 Analysing Changes and Differences in EQ-5D Values and EQ VAS Scores

In the analyses described in Chaps. 3 and 4, the objects of interest are EQ-5D values or EQ VAS scores measured at one or more points in time for one person or a group of people. These can be compared between the same person at different time points, which we will call 'changes', or between different people or groups of people, which we will call 'differences.' When the object of interest is the change or difference itself, analysts should be cautious in the way that they deal with them.

5.1.1 Defining the Outcome of an Intervention Study as a Change

In clinical studies of the impact of a health care intervention on health-related quality of life (HRQoL), it is possible to define the outcome in two different ways—the

N. Devlin et al., *Methods for Analysing and Reporting EQ-5D Data*,
https://doi.org/10.1007/978-3-030-47622-9_5

final state of health or the change from initial to final state. In many contexts, the magnitude as well as direction of the change is the object of interest, but there are some well-known issues about estimating the size of changes directly. These relate to all outcome measures, not just health status or HRQoL (for example Vickers and Altman 2001; Bland and Altman 2011), and to Patient Reported Outcome Measures (PROMs) other than EQ-5D instruments, but the characteristics of EQ-5D and EQ VAS values data mean that they are particularly vulnerable to misleading analysis through misspecification of the underlying analytical model.

The key issue is the relationship between the size of initial, or baseline, health state values and the size of the change in them. The most obvious null hypothesis is that baseline and final mean HRQoL scores are the same, equivalent to a mean change score of zero. However, for conditions where underlying health is deteriorating or the condition is self-limiting, this null hypothesis may not be the correct choice. The size of the change may also be related to the baseline in different ways, depending on both the condition and the treatment. For example, if the treatment leads to the same final health state for all patients, the change will be greater, the lower the initial health state; if the treatment is less successful for those with a poorer health state, the change will be greater, the higher the initial health state. Only if the change is constant whatever the initial health state will there be no such complicating relationship.

Figure 5.1 illustrates this point. The horizontal and vertical axes show baseline and final EQ 5D values scores respectively. The solid 45° line shows points where baseline and final are the same, which would be the null hypothesis for patients whose condition is neither improving or deteriorating. The dotted line shows a different

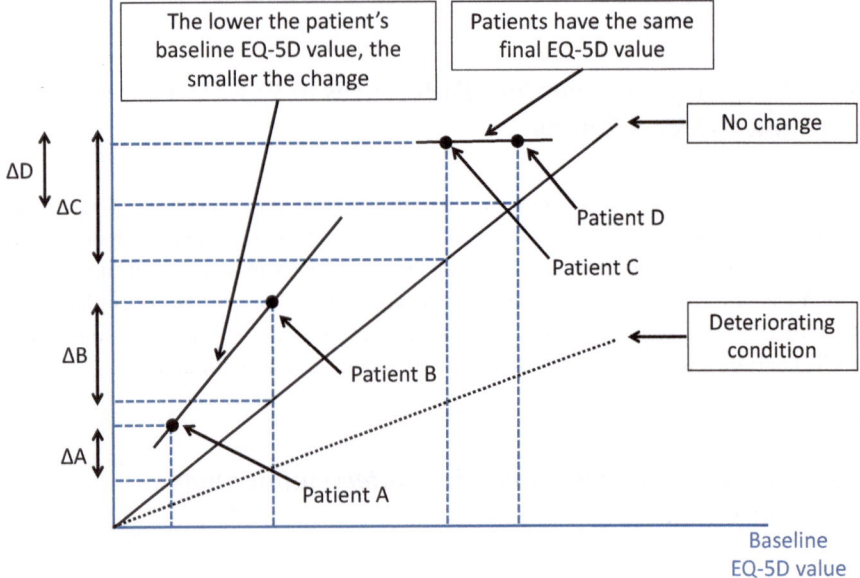

Fig. 5.1 Stylised example of treatment effects

assumption: that the condition would result in a deterioration of the patients' health over time if untreated. The two solid lines above the 'No Change' line show different relationships between baseline and final scores for two different treatments. Patients A and B undergo a treatment for which the outcomes are better for patients whose baseline score is higher. Assuming the null hypothesis of no improvement or deterioration without treatment, the change after treatment for patient A, who has a lower baseline score than patient B, is smaller (ΔA) than that for patient B (ΔB). Patients C and D undergo a treatment which results in the same final score for all patients. Again, assuming that there would be no change without treatment, the change for patient C, who has a lower baseline score than patient D, is bigger (ΔC) than that for patient D (ΔD).

The special problem that this raises for both EQ-5D values and EQ VAS scores is that the existence of fixed end-points—0 and 100 for the EQ VAS; 1 and the value of the worst health state for EQ-5D values—places limits on the possible size of change. (The same is true for any outcome measure that has the same properties.) For EQ-5D values, there is an additional problem that the distribution of scores at both baseline and final assessment may not be smooth because of the discrete nature of the EQ-5D health states from which the scores are calculated. These two issues also mean that there may not be the necessary linear relationship between the baseline and final outcome scores that would permit calculation of a single change-based effect size.

The recommendations are therefore to specify carefully the counterfactual to the observed change or difference, or where possible to ensure that there are control groups from which this can be directly measured, and to ensure that appropriate methods are used to transform the distribution of EQ-5D values into a form amenable to statistical analysis.

5.1.2   Minimal Important Differences (MIDs)

The calculation of Minimal Important Differences (MIDs) for HRQoL or PRO measures, including the EQ-5D, is a topic on which there is currently no consensus, either to its usefulness or the best methods for its estimation. Those who wish to use or estimate MIDs are therefore advised to consult two review articles, one on MIDs in general (King 2011) and the other specifically on the EQ-5D (Coretti et al. 2014). Here we summarise some of the issues.

The term MID is used here, but other terms are used which, as King points out, may differ slightly in their definitions and meaning such as *minimal clinically important difference (MCID), clinically important difference, minimally detectable difference, minimum detectable change,* and *subjectively significant difference.* The most widely quoted definition of the concept is of a MCID (Jaeschke et al. 1989), but an updated MID-specific version of this (Guyatt et al. 2002) is "the smallest difference in score in the domain of interest that patients perceive as important, either beneficial or harmful, and which would lead the clinician to consider a change in the patient's management". Coretti et al. make use of a different term, *the smallest worthwhile effect* (SWE), defined by Ferreira et al. (2012) as "the smallest beneficial effect justifying costs, risks and inconveniences of an intervention."

There are three key questions to address when deciding whether and how to use MIDs with an HRQoL or PRO measure such as the EQ-5D: What is the purpose of using a MID? What definition should be used for that purpose? and How should the MID be estimated to meet that definition? Although in principle it would be possible to ask these questions about EQ-5D health states, in practice they have only been explored for EQ-5D values and to a lesser extent to EQ VAS scores, so this guide has the same limitation.

In answering these questions, it is essential to note that EQ-5D values have a feature that distinguishes them from some other measures. They already embody a measure of importance as perceived by a group of people, usually a general population, based on their preferences for different health states (see Chap. 4). The values are estimated from an underlying continuous value function at discrete points on the value scale identified by the EQ-5D health states. Any differences in the underlying values, however small, are therefore important in that they indicate a difference that would be preferred or non-preferred by the person affected, other things being equal. Similar arguments apply to the scores generated by the EQ VAS.

A wider definition of importance, such as whether a change is worthwhile given the perceived importance to patients and resource costs of making the change and the duration for which the change is experienced, requires information that is not contained within the EQ-5D values or EQ VAS scores themselves. This suggests that there is no conceptual basis for a MID for EQ-5D values or EQ VAS scores in terms of *desirability*; however, it may be possible to base a MID on whether in practice differences and changes in the EQ-5D values or EQ VAS score are *detectable*. As King points out, this concept of 'minimally detectable' differences or changes has two separate bases. One is psychometric, and concerns whether a difference is capable of being perceived by people. The other is statistical, concerning measurement error, the precision with which perceived differences are recorded.

Using EQ-5D MIDs

Using EQ-5D MIDs for decision making with individual patients

As noted, the basis for an EQ-5D MID to judge the importance, in terms of desirability, of differences between or changes in health states is weak. A further problem for using this with individual patients is that they may not share the preferences of the average patient or member of the general population about their health. With respect to detectability, the ability to observe changes or differences in EQ-5D values is entirely based on detection of changes to the EQ-5D health states, and the calculation of a summary index in the form of an EQ-5D value may obscure rather than illuminate the nature of the change.

Using EQ-5D MIDs for decision making about populations

Again, it is not possible to judge, in terms of desirability, whether an observed difference or change in EQ-5D values or EQ VAS scores is important without further information. With respect to detectability, there is also a problem arising from how observations for individual people are aggregated to give a population score, exacerbated in the case of the EQ-5D values by their discrete nature. A population average MID will depend both on the size of changes to each individual person's health state and the number of people experiencing different levels of change. As an extreme example, if all but one member of a group recorded a change of EQ-5D values at the MID value and the exception scored below that, the population would be judged as having a difference below the MID. Comparing the mean to the MID would give a misleading account of the clinical importance of the overall observed differences.

Using EQ-5D MIDs for clinical research

A proposed use of MIDs is in determining the most efficient sample size for a clinical trial, based on the desired probabilities of avoiding type 1 and type 2 errors. The aim is to ensure that trials are not over-powered, and generate statistically significant differences that have no clinical significance. A trial powered to detect differences at the level of the MID would be the correct approach for a trial for which HRQoL was the primary endpoint and was the sole determinant of clinical decision making. However, the MID is less useful for trials that have a different primary endpoint or where clinical decision making is not independent of factors other than a difference in HRQoL. In addition, it is again necessary to take account of the distribution of observed differences in EQ-5D values, as using an individually-based MID may be misleading about the total benefit over all patients.

MID estimation methods

A common finding of the different methods described below is that there is no identifiable single MID for EQ-5D values or EQ VAS scores. Instead, estimates differ by population, patient group, clinical context and sociodemographic factors; and might vary depending on whether health is improving or worsening. It is possible to calculate a score which is an average over different patient populations, such as the widely-quoted estimate by Walters and Brazier (2005) for EQ-5D values (which is described below), but although this is an interesting statistic, the size of the variability between different estimates means that an average EQ-5D MID should not be used for any of the purposes described above.

Patient rating of change

The most common and direct method of meeting the aim of assessing patients' own perceptions of the importance of differences in their health is to quiz them specifically about that, using a *global transition question*. This is a retrospective assessment by patients of the change in their health between two points, at each of which their current health has been assessed using the HRQoL or PRO instrument. For example, Walters and Brazier (2005) re-analysed 11 studies in different clinical areas that collected both EQ-5D and SF-36 data at different time points. They compared the differences between EQ-5D values with a question taken from the SF-36, asking if their general health was much better, somewhat better, stayed the same, somewhat worse or much worse, compared to the last time they were assessed. Those who answered somewhat better or somewhat worse were considered as having experienced a change equivalent to the MID.

This method relies on the global transition question identifying the minimum perception that patients can have, which is in reality determined by the fixed wording of the text of the permitted answers. For example, patients are likely to have different thresholds for deciding that they have any improvement or deterioration at all, and also different perceptions of the boundaries between 'somewhat' and 'much'. If these do not match the boundaries between the descriptions contained in the EQ-5D health states, then the calculated EQ-5D value changes for the 'somewhat' categories may not reflect the true size of the minimum differences that patients perceive. In addition, global transition questions are affected by the ability of patients to recall their previous health state accurately and may be more subject to acquiescence bias and response shift (Sprangers and Schwartz 1999; Kamper et al. 2009).

Clinical anchors

Another common method of defining a MID is to examine the scores of patients classified according to a different measure of their clinical status. The rationale is that for clinical decision making, clinicians may have more confidence with an HRQoL measure if it is related to more familiar, clinically-focussed and well-validated measures. For example, Pickard et al. (2007) calculated the mean EQ-5D values and EQ VAS scores for cancer patients in the different grades of two clinical measures, the Eastern Cancer Oncology Group (ECOG) and the Functional Assessment of Cancer Therapy General (FACT-G). The differences between the mean scores between different grades, ordered according to severity of the condition, provides MID estimates as a range and average.

This method emphasises the clinical decision-making aspect of the definition of a MID rather than the idea that it should reflect patients' own perception of the importance of change. It therefore depends on an assumption that the clinical anchor measure correctly distinguishes between important and unimportant changes in health states.

Distribution-based

Some estimates of the MID are based on statistics that describe the distribution of health states in a patient population, in particular the standard error of measurement (SEM) and the effect size (ES). Pickard et al. (2007) also estimated MIDs for EQ-5D values and EQ VAS scores using both of these approaches, stratified again according to FACT-G and ECOG grades. The SEM is based on reliability of the HRQoL or PRO instrument, usually measured with respect to test-retest reliability, the distribution around a true score of repeated assessments assuming no memory effect or other contextual changes, which is regarded as a fixed psychometric property of the instrument. An alternative measure is reliability based on internal consistency measured by Cronbach's alpha, which is what Pickard et al. used because of the scarcity of test-retest information for the EQ-5D.

The ES is calculated as the mean difference in HRQoL divided by the between-person standard deviation. Pickard et al. based their MIDs on the criterion of one-half of the standard deviation (SD), although one-third and one-fifth SD are also commonly used (King 2011).

These methods again do not reflect patients' perceptions of importance, and unless they are stratified in the way used by Pickard et al. also do not reflect importance as defined by a clinician for use in decision-making.

Instrument-defined

Luo et al. (2010) and McClure et al. (2017) have calculated MIDs for the 3L and 5L respectively using a method that does not require empirical EQ-5D or other data. It is calculated, for a specified value set, as the smallest difference in the values of any pair of health states, over all possible pairs. It is therefore the smallest possible observed difference in values either for a person whose EQ-5D health state is captured at two different times or for two people at the same time.

This highlights an important property of a value set, and is useful in examining the comparative performance of different value sets. However, it does not match with the usual definitions of a MID and it is not obvious how it might be used for any of the purposes described above. The differences between the values of different health states are entirely determined by perceived differences in the descriptions that the health states are given. This MID therefore does not reflect the smallest score that people find important, but the smallest difference between the health state descriptions, which is fixed by the descriptive system itself, not by the people who value them. As importantly, it is based on an assessment of health state differences for individual people, and in a group or population context, it is highly vulnerable to the problem outlined above of the mean giving a misleading account of overall clinical importance.

The overall recommendation for MIDs is that the purpose of using a MID in a particular context should be carefully considered, that a precise definition for the MID is derived from that purpose, and that the methods used to estimate that MID fit with the definition adopted.

5.1.3 Case-Mix and Risk Adjustment of EQ-5D Data

Although we refer here to case-mix adjustment, the principles also apply to the related concept of risk adjustment. Adjusting HRQoL or PRO scores for the differing characteristics of patients and external factors is often essential in making comparisons of outcomes. For example, when comparing the average observed EQ-5D value or EQ VAS score changes after treatment for patients in different hospitals, it is important to account for factors that affect outcomes but are not due to variations in the quality of care. One such factor may be the average age of patients treated, which may differ between different providers and affect the outcomes that can be achieved. To obtain a fair comparison of the outcomes of different hospitals, they should be adjusted to take account of the mix of cases that the hospitals see.

There are many different methods for calculating case-mix adjustments, including stratification and direct and indirect standardisation. Stratification refers to calculation of outcomes for subgroups of a population defined according to key characteristics that might affect outcomes, such as age, sex and ethnicity. Direct standardisation calculates outcomes for different units, such as hospitals, adjusted by comparison of the levels of the case-mix variables to those in a known reference population. Indirect standardisation uses, instead of a known reference population, the average level of the variables for the units as a whole. Here we give an example of how the United Kingdom's National Health Service (NHS) adjusts for case-mix in its PROMs programme (Nuttall et al. 2015; Department of Health 2012; NHS England Analytical Team 2013) using the indirect standardisation method.

The NHS case-mix adjustment method has two stages. The average impact of case-mix variables on EQ-5D values or EQ VAS scores is calculated over all patients using regression analysis. The regression coefficients are used to estimate, for each health care provider, the average EQ-5D value or EQ VAS score that would be expected for its mix of those variables. From this, the difference between expected and actual outcomes is calculated for each provider.

This is regarded as a measure of a provider's performance, but the 'expected' outcome is for a hypothetical provider that has the same case-mix, and does not compare the provider with other real providers. Each provider's outcomes are therefore transformed so that they can be compared to a standard case-mix, which is the mean level of the case-mix variables over all providers. This also generates the all-providers average EQ-5D value or EQ VAS score, by definition.

Figure 5.2 illustrates this, using a very simple case-mix adjustment to the post-treatment EQ-5D value or EQ VAS score (Q2), taking account of the pre-treatment value of the score (Q1). An observation on the Q1 = Q2 line would mean that there had been no change in the average EQ-5D value or EQ VAS score. The hypothetical regression line lies above this, meaning that at all levels of Q1 there is on average an improvement following surgery. Q2 is higher with higher Q1, but the size of the improvement (the difference between Q2 and Q1) is smaller with higher Q1.

For provider A, its average post-surgery EQ-5D value or EQ VAS score is Q2a, so that the change in the EQ-5D value or EQ VAS score unadjusted for case-mix is ΔQ = Q2a−Q1a. Its expected EQ-5D value or EQ VAS score is Q2b and it therefore has performed better than would be expected for a provider that had the same case-mix.

Performance can be quantified as Q2a−Q2b; if this is positive, the provider achieves on average results greater than those predicted; negative if worse than predicted; and zero if as predicted. This difference is applied to the all-provider Q2 EQ-5D value or EQ VAS score, which is Q2d, to give the estimated actual EQ-5D value or EQ VAS score for Provider A if it had the all-provider case-mix. This EQ-5D value or EQ VAS score, Q2c, is calculated so that Q2c−Q2d = Q2a−Q2b, which means Q2c = Q2d + (Q2a−Q2b). The relevant Q1 comparator for this is the all-provider Q1 EQ-5D value or EQ VAS score, so the case-mix adjusted change in the EQ-5D value or EQ VAS score for Provider A is $\Delta Q'$ = Q2c−Q1.

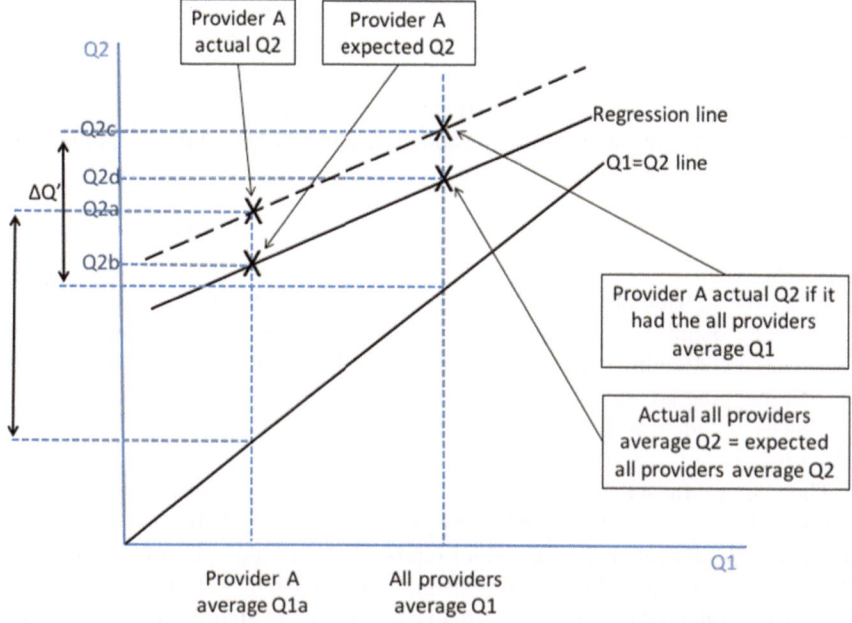

Fig. 5.2 Stylised example of case-mix adjustment. This figure is taken from Chapter 3 of Appleby et al. (2015)

Amongst the problems with this method are those outlined in Sect. 5.1.1 concerning the assumed counterfactual to the observed changes and the effect of fixed end-points and discrete EQ-5D values on the distribution of changes and their relationship with the pre-surgery EQ-5D values or EQ VAS scores.

Case-mix adjustments can change the estimated outcomes for different units such that a very different assessment is made of their relative performance. For example, Appleby et al. (2015) showed that using a case-mix adjustment for changes in EQ-5D values in the English NHS PROMs programme reduced the range of average hospital scores and the size of their variability around the national average. More importantly, it produces a different performance ranking of hospitals in terms of health gain, as individual hospitals' adjusted and unadjusted gains differ considerably in many cases.

5.2 Mapping

In this context, mapping refers to methods that are used to convert the responses of one HRQoL or PRO measure to those of a different measure. The most usual application for the EQ-5D is based on an interpretation of EQ-5D values as numbers representing the values that people attach to health states, which have cardinal measurement properties such that they can be used to calculate Quality Adjusted Life Years, which can be used as the denominator in an Incremental Cost Effectiveness Ratio. Mapping is used to convert data from a measure that does not have these properties, such as a condition specific instrument, to EQ-5D values. This takes the form of an algorithm which is applied to the source measure and generates EQ-5D values. Mapping could also be used simply to translate the responses given in another HRQOL measure into EQ-5D health states.

Mapping is also used to convert between the values of the 3L and 5L versions. However, we will not discuss the methods used for this as they concern valuation of health states, which is outside of the scope of this review. At the time of writing, there are no definitive guidelines for those who wish to convert 3L to 5L or vice versa, and a continuing debate about the best methods. Those wishing to make use of such mapping are advised to consult the most up-to-date literature; current key references include van Hout et al. (2012), Hernandez-Alava et al. (2017) and Dakin et al. (2018).

There are useful statements of good practice in mapping to health state measures that have the value-based and cardinality properties described above from measures that do not (Wailoo et al. 2017), and for reporting those studies (Petrou et al. 2015). There is also an online database of existing mapping studies (Dakin 2013). Those who wish to undertake mapping or use existing mapping algorithms are advised to consult those papers, and here we simply summarise some of the issues. It should be emphasised that mapping is a second-best approach that produces only an approximation to true EQ-5D values. The availability of a mapping algorithm for a particular measure can never be a justification for failing to collect EQ-5D health state data as well as or instead of that measure.

The earliest studies that undertook mapping were often based on direct judgements by clinical experts, patients or researchers about the correspondence between the descriptive systems of the source measure and EQ-5D values. This is not now regarded as good practice. Acceptable mapping methods require data that have been collected from respondents who have completed both the source measure and the EQ-5D.

There is a broad division of mapping methods between those that map directly to EQ-5D values and those, known as *response mapping*, that map to EQ-5D health states, from which EQ-5D values are calculated using a value set. For the direct method, it is possible simply to assign EQ-5D values for the health state recorded by each respondent to the category or score that they report for the source measure, and calculate the mean over all respondents. However, this method is restrictive, because it only enables mapping for those health states present in the sample in large enough numbers. It is also known that other patient characteristics and health and treatment condition variables may impact on the mapping. As a result, it is regarded as best practice to use a regression-based method to ensure that the mapping algorithm is both more comprehensive and more precise.

The response mapping method has the advantage, when *using* a mapping algorithm, that it produces an algorithm that generates EQ-5D health states, to which any value set can be applied, while the direct method is specific to a particular value set.

The direct method has the advantage, when *generating* a mapping algorithm, that in estimating the relationship between the source measure and the EQ-5D, the response or dependent variable—EQ-5D values—can be treated as a continuous variable. The response mapping method is based on categories—EQ-5D health states—that do not even have ordinal properties. This is a problem because it potentially requires a data set large enough to contain a meaningfully-large observation for each of the 243 (3L) or 3125 (5L) health states. However, in practice this problem is dealt with by assuming that the level recorded in each dimension is independent of the level recorded in other dimensions. This permits estimation of five separate ordered dependent variables, which is statistically much more amenable to analysis.

References

Appleby J, Devlin N, Parkin D (2015) Using patient reported outcomes to improve health care. Wiley Blackwell

Bland JM, Altman DG (2011) Comparisons against baseline within randomised groups are often used and can be highly misleading. Trials 12(1):264

Coretti S, Ruggeri M, McNamee P (2014) The minimum clinically important difference for EQ-5D index: a critical review. Expert Rev Pharmacoecon Outcomes Res 14(2):221–233

Dakin H (2013) Review of studies mapping from quality of life or clinical measures to EQ-5D: an online database. Health Qual Life Outcomes 11:151

Dakin H, Abel L, Burns R, Yang Y (2018) Review and critical appraisal of studies mapping from quality of life or clinical measures to EQ-5D: an online database and application of the MAPS statement. Health Qual Life Outcomes 16(1):31

Department of Health (2012) Patient Reported Outcome Measures (PROMs) in England: The case-mix adjustment methodology. London: Department of Health

Ferreira ML, Herbert RD, Ferreira PH et al (2012) A critical review of methods used to determine the smallest worthwhile effect of interventions for low back pain. J Clin Epidemiol 65(3):253–61

Guyatt GH, Osaba D, Wu AW et al (2002) Methods to explain the clinical significance of health status measures. Mayo Clin Proc 77(4):371–383

Hernandez Alava M, Wailoo A, Pudney S (2017) Methods for mapping between the EQ-5D-5L and the 3L for technology appraisal: report by the NICE Decision Support Unit. School of Health and Related Research, University of Sheffield, UK, Health Economics and Decision Science

van Hout B, Janssen MF, Feng Y et al (2012) Interim scoring for the EQ-5D-5L: mapping the EQ-5D-5L to EQ-5D-3L value sets. Value Health 15:708–15

Jaeschke R, Singer J, Guyatt GH (1989) Measurement of health status: ascertaining the minimal clinically important difference. Control Clin Trials 10(4):407–15

Kamper SJ, Maher CG, Mackay G (2009) Global rating of change scales: a review of strengths and weaknesses and considerations for design. J Man Manip Ther 17(3):163–70

King MT (2011) A point of minimal important difference (MID): a critique of terminology and methods. Expert Rev Pharmacoecon Outcomes Res 11(2):171–184

Luo N, Johnson JA, Coons SJ (2010) Using instrument-defined health state transitions to estimate minimally important differences for four preference-based health-related quality of life instruments. Med Care 48:365–71

McClure NS, Al Sayah F, Xie F, Luo N, Johnson JA (2017) Instrument-defined estimates of the minimally important difference for EQ-5D-5L index scores. Value Health 20:644–650

NHS England Analytical Team (2013) Patient Reported Outcome Measures (PROMs): An alternative aggregation methodology for case-mix adjustment. NHS England. http://www.england.nhs.uk/statistics/wp-content/uploads/sites/2/2013/07/proms-agg-meth-adju.pdf

Nuttall D, Parkin D, Devlin N (2015) Inter-provider comparison of patient-reported outcomes: developing an adjustment to account for differences in patient case mix. Health Econ 24(1):41–54

Petrou S, Rivero-Arias O, Dakin H, Longworth L, Oppe M, Froud R, Gray A (2015) The MAPS reporting statement for studies mapping onto generic preference-based outcome measures: explanation and elaboration. PharmacoEconomics 33:993–1011

Pickard AS, Neary MP, Cella D (2007) Estimation of minimally important differences in EQ-5D utility and VAS scores in cancer. Health Qual Life Outcomes 5:70

Sprangers MA, Schwartz CE (1999) Integrating response shift into health-related quality of life research: a theoretical model. Soc Sci Med 48:1507–1515

Vickers AJ, Altman DG (2001) Analysing controlled trials with baseline and follow up measurements. BMJ 323(7321):1123–1124

Wailoo AJ, Hernandez-Alava M, Manca A, Mejia A, Ray J, Crawford B, Botteman M, Busschbach J (2017) Mapping to estimate health-state utility from non–preference-based outcome measures: an ISPOR good practices for outcomes research task force report. Value Health 20:18–27

Walters SJ, Brazier JE (2005) Comparison of the minimally important difference for two health state utility measures: EQ-5D and SF-6D. Qual Life Res 14:32

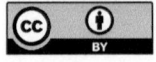

Glossary of EQ-5D Terms

In this section, we set out the terms used in this book to describe specific aspects of the EQ-5D instruments. It is important to use these terms consistently in papers and reports, as this ensures effective communication and avoids confusion between terms that have very different meanings. For example, the visual analogue scale element of the EQ-5D questionnaire, which is used to report a respondent's overall current health state, should not be confused with a visual analogue scale used as a stated preference method for valuing defined EQ-5D health states. The first is therefore called the EQ VAS and the second the EQ-5D VAS.

Term	Description
EQ-5D	The family of instruments developed and maintained by the EuroQol Group, currently the EQ-5D-3L, the EQ-5D-5L and the EQ-5D-Y
EQ-5D-3L	Refers to either the EQ-5D-3L descriptive system or the EQ-5D-3L questionnaire 'EQ-5D-3L' should always be referred to in full at first usage, but thereafter can be shortened to '3L'
EQ-5D-3L descriptive system	Descriptive system for health-related quality of life states consisting of five dimensions (Mobility, Self-care, Usual activities, Pain & discomfort, Anxiety & depression), each of which has three severity levels that are described by statements appropriate to that dimension
EQ-5D-3L questionnaire	Standard layout for recording a person's current self-reported health state. Consists of a standard format for respondents to record their health state according to the EQ-5D-3L descriptive system and the EQ VAS
EQ-5D-5L	Refers to either the EQ-5D-5L descriptive system or the EQ-5D-5L questionnaire 'EQ-5D-5L' should always be referred to in full at first usage, but thereafter can be shortened to '5L'

(continued)

© The Author(s) 2020
N. Devlin et al., *Methods for Analysing and Reporting EQ-5D Data*,
https://doi.org/10.1007/978-3-030-47622-9

(continued)

Term	Description
EQ-5D-5L descriptive system	Descriptive system for health-related quality of life states consisting of five dimensions (Mobility, Self-care, Usual activities, Pain & discomfort, Anxiety & depression), each of which has five severity levels that are described by statements appropriate to that dimension
EQ-5D-5L questionnaire	Standard layout for recording a person's current self-reported health state. Consists of a standard format for respondents to record their health state according to the EQ-5D-5L descriptive system and the EQ VAS
EQ-5D-Y	The Youth version of the EQ-5D, suitable for younger people. Refers either to the EQ-5D-Y descriptive system or the EQ-5D-Y questionnaire An expanded level version of the EQ-5D-Y is currently being developed. Once this is completed, the current version of the EQ-5D-Y will become the EQ-5D-Y-3L
EQ-5D-Y descriptive system	Descriptive system for young peoples' health-related quality of life states consisting of five dimensions (Mobility, Looking after myself, Doing usual activities, Having pain or discomfort, Feeling worried, sad or unhappy), each of which has three severity levels that are described by statements appropriate to that dimension
EQ-5D-Y questionnaire	Standard layout for recording a young person's current self-reported health state. Consists of a standard format for respondents to record their health state according to the EQ-5D-Y descriptive system and the EQ VAS
EQ-5D proxy questionnaires	A questionnaire that records a person's current health state as rated by a caregiver who knows the person well. Consists of a standard format for the proxy to record the person's health state according to the relevant EQ-5D descriptive system and the EQ VAS
EQ VAS	A standard vertical 20 cm visual analogue scale, used in recording an individual's rating of their overall current health-related quality of life. The scale ranges from 100 ('the best imaginable health state' or 'the best health state you can imagine') to 0 ('the worst imaginable health state' or 'the worst health you can imagine') There are different versions of these for the EQ-5D-3L, the EQ-5D-5L and the EQ-5D-Y; these are currently being harmonised. In the 5L, Y and harmonised versions, the scale is accompanied by a box to record the rating
EQ-5D profile	A description of a health state defined by one of the EQ-5D descriptive systems. This may be summarised by a series of five sentences, one for each dimension and stating the level within that dimension; or a label consisting of five ordinal numbers, one for each dimension (by convention, in the order these appear in the questionnaire), defining the severity level, where 1 means no problems

(continued)

(continued)

Term	Description
EQ-5D self-reported health state	A health state recorded by a respondent using any of the EQ-5D questionnaires or by an interviewer recording their responses on the questionnaire. This may be summarised in the same way as the EQ-5D profile
EQ-5D proxy-reported health state	A health state recorded by a proxy acting for the person experiencing it using any of the EQ-5D proxy questionnaires. This may be summarised in the same way as the EQ-5D profile
EQ VAS score	Score between 0 and 100 recorded by an individual for their current overall health-related quality of life using the EQ VAS
EQ-5D values	The value attached to an EQ-5D profile according to a set of weights that reflect, on average, people's preferences about how good or bad the state is. Values are anchored at 1 (full health) and 0 (a state as bad as being dead) as required by their use in economic evaluation. Values less than 0 represent health states regarded as worse than a state that is as bad as being dead An EQ-5D value is also sometimes known as an 'index', 'score' or 'utility'
EQ-5D value set	A list of the value for every possible EQ-5D profile within a given descriptive system. For example, a value set for the EQ-5D-5L shows a value for each of the 3125 states that are described by it. These values are usually calculated using an algorithm that assigns a score to each level in each dimension, sometimes including adjustments for interactions between the dimensions As value sets represent the average values of a sample of people, for example the general public of a particular country, it is important to state which value set is being used Value sets are also sometimes referred to as 'tariffs'
EQ-VT	The EuroQol Valuation Technology. Software developed by the EuroQol Group to obtain values for the EQ-5D in computer-assisted personal interviews. The methods currently used in EQ-VT to obtain stated preferences for EQ-5D health states are time trade-off (TTO) and discrete choice experiments (DCE)
EQ-5D valuation questionnaire	Questionnaire, of standard layout, consisting of the EQ-5D questionnaire plus the EQ-5D VAS for a selection of EQ-5D profiles, and a standard set of instructions The EQ-5D valuation questionnaire was used in early research to value EQ-5D-3 and is now rarely used. Descriptions of it and its components are included here for completeness and clarity

(continued)

(continued)

Term	Description
EQ-5D VAS	Visual analogue scale, of standard 20 cm layout, for recording an individual's valuation of defined EQ-5D profiles. The scale ranges from 100 ('the best imaginable health state' or 'the best health state you can imagine') to 0 ('the worst imaginable health state' or 'the worst health you can imagine'). This is used to obtain a respondent's stated preference values, not to record their own health state
EQ-5D VAS value	Stated preference score recorded by an individual for an EQ-5D profile using the EQ-5D VAS